BRIGHT FUTURES

NUTRITION

THIRD EDITION

POCKET GUIDE

Katrina Holt, MPH, MS, RD

Editor

PUBLISHED BY

American Academy of Pediatrics

American Academy of Pediatrics Department of Marketing and Publications Staff

Maureen DeRosa, MPA
Director, Department of Marketing and Publications

Mark Grimes
Director, Division of Product Development

Sandi King, MS
Director, Division of Publishing and Production Services

Maryjo Reynolds
Product Manager, Bright Futures

Peg Mulcahy
Manager, Graphic Design and Production

Kate Larson
Manager, Editorial Services

Kevin Tuley
Director, Division of Marketing and Sales

Bright Futures: Nutrition, 3rd Edition Pocket Guide
Library of Congress Control Number: 2010917945
ISBN: 978-1-58110-555-1
Product Code: BF0038

The recommendations in this publication do not indicate an exclusive course of treatment or serve as a standard of care. Variations, taking into account individual circumstances, may be appropriate.

Every effort has been made to ensure that the drug selection and dosage set forth in this text are in accordance with the current recommendations and practice at the time of the publication. It is the responsibility of the health care provider to check the package insert of each drug for any change in indications or dosage and for added warnings and precautions.

The mention of product names in this publication is for informational purposes only and does not imply endorsement by the American Academy of Pediatrics.

This publication has been produced by the American Academy of Pediatrics under its cooperative agreement (U04MC07853) with the US Department of Health and Human Services, Health Resources and Services Administration (HRSA), Maternal and Child Health Bureau (MCHB).

1 2 3 4 5 6 7 8 9 10

TABLE OF CONTENTS

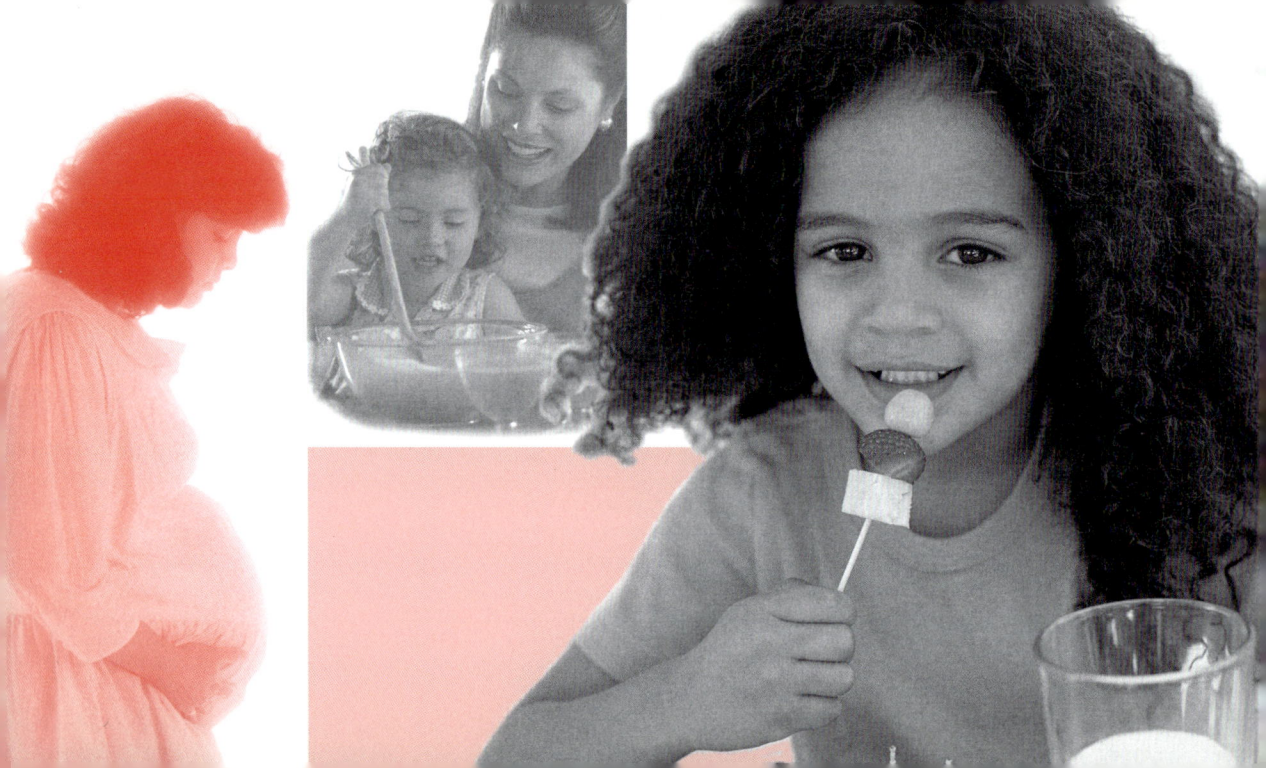

Bright Futures: Nutrition

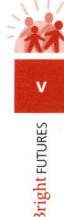

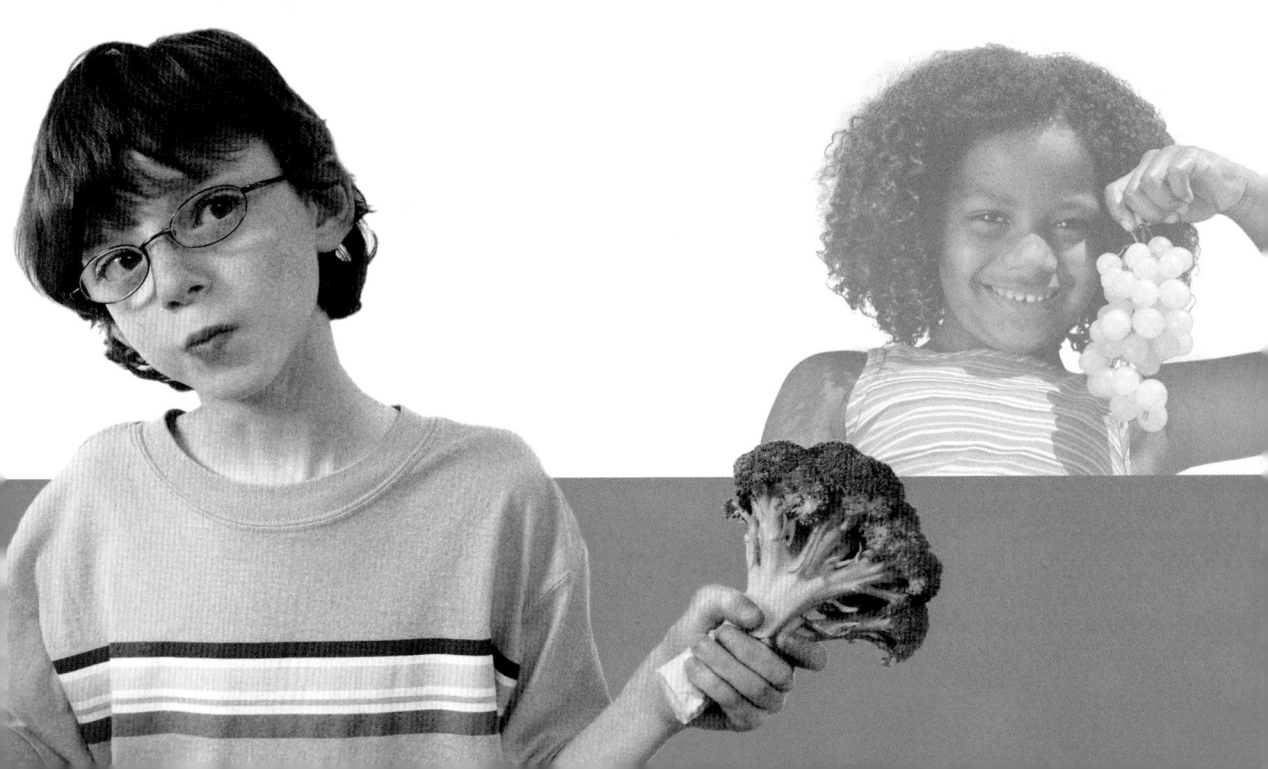

BUILDING *BRIGHT FUTURES: NUTRITION*

*B*right Futures: Nutrition is offered in the spirit of health promotion. This comprehensive guide is based on 3 critical principles consistent with the Bright Futures conceptual framework

1. Nutrition must be integrated into the lives of infants, children, adolescents, and families.
2. Good nutrition requires balance.
3. An element of joy enhances nutrition, health, and well-being.

Bright Futures: Nutrition weaves nutrition principles into all aspects of daily life. It incorporates a clear understanding that food availability, family and cultural customs, and external social pressures (eg, those created by the media) all influence infants, children's, and adolescents' eating behaviors. Integrating good nutrition into the lives of infants, children, and adolescents requires effort in many settings: the home, child care facilities, the school system, and the community.

Balance is central to good nutrition and good health: the balance of calories, protein, fat, carbohydrates, vitamins, and minerals in the diet; the balance of dependence and independence between the parent and the infant, child, or adolescent; and the balance of cultural norms and secular trends. *Bright Futures: Nutrition* describes ways in which food and nutrition can be balanced for good health.

A sense of joy of is fundamental to the effective integration of healthy nutrition into people's lives. The contributors to *Bright Futures: Nutrition* value the sense of wonder and joy in infants, children, adolescents, families, and communities. Nutrition planning and preparing and sharing food are seen as happy events that bring people together—the infant at the mother's breast, the family at the dinner table, and the community at the clam bake.

Bright Futures: Nutrition provides a thorough overview of nutrition supervision during infancy, early childhood, middle childhood, and adolescence. We hope that the guide's emphasis on nutritional integration, balance, and joy will improve the lives of infants, children, adolescents, and their families.

vii

BRIGHT FUTURES: NUTRITION VISION AND GOALS

The vision and goals of *Bright Futures: Nutrition* are to

- Improve the nutrition status of infants, children, and adolescents.
- Identify desired health and nutrition outcomes that result from positive nutrition status.
- Set guidelines to help health professionals promote the nutrition status of infants, children, and adolescents.
- Encourage partnerships among health professionals, families, and communities to promote the nutrition status of infants, children, and adolescents.
- Describe the roles of health professionals in delivering nutrition services within the community.
- Identify opportunities for coordination and collaboration between health professionals and the community.

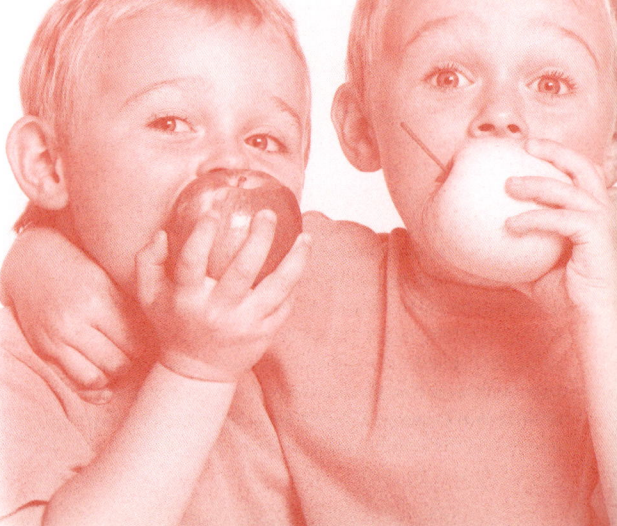

ABOUT *BRIGHT FUTURES: NUTRITION*

A Developmental and Contextual Approach

Bright Futures: Nutrition represents a developmental and contextual approach for helping infants, children, and adolescents develop positive attitudes toward food and practice healthy eating behaviors.

The developmental approach, which is based on the unique social and psychological characteristics of each developmental period, is critical for understanding infants, children's, and adolescents' attitudes toward food and for encouraging healthy eating behaviors.

The contextual approach emphasizes the promotion of positive attitudes toward food and healthy eating behaviors by providing infants, children, adolescents, and their families with consistent nutrition messages. Consistency, combined with flexibility, is essential for handling the challenges of infancy and early childhood. During middle childhood and adolescence, it is important for parents to encourage their children and adolescents to become more responsible for their own health and to help them develop the skills they need to practice healthy eating behaviors.

Bright Futures: Nutrition recommends that food and eating be viewed as both health-enhancing and pleasurable. Food provides more than just energy and sustenance. It holds innumerable symbolic, emotional, social, and personal meanings. Food is connected with nurturing, family, culture, tradition, and celebration. Promoting positive attitudes toward food and healthy eating behaviors in infants, children, and adolescents involves recognizing the multiple meanings of food and creating an environment that encourages the enjoyment of food. Family meals are emphasized because they help build on family strengths and promote unity, social bonds, and good communication.

Partnerships Among Health Professionals, Families, and Communities

Encouraging healthy eating behaviors in infants, children, and adolescents is a shared responsibility. One of the principles of *Bright Futures: Nutrition* is that, together, health professionals, families, and communities can make a difference in the nutrition status of infants, children, and adolescents.

Today many families face the challenges of balancing work and home life and dealing with hectic schedules. Health professionals can help families learn how to fit nutritious meals and snacks into their busy lives. To be most effective, strategies need to be tailored to the family's individual needs.

The family is the predominant influence on infants', children's, and adolescents' attitudes toward food and their adoption of healthy eating behaviors. The family exerts this influence by

- Providing food
- Transmitting attitudes, preferences, and values about food, which affect lifetime eating behaviors
- Establishing the social environment in which food is shared

Parents want to know how they can contribute to their infants', children's, and adolescents' health and are looking for guidance; however, they are faced with contradictory nutrition information. Dietary recommendations can be misunderstood or misinterpreted, especially when adult guidelines are applied to children and adolescents.

Throughout the nutrition pocket guide, we use the term "parent" to refer to the adult or adults responsible for the care of the infant, child, or adolescent. In some situations this person could be an aunt, uncle, grandparent, custodian, or legal guardian.

The community can be invaluable in helping children and adolescents develop positive attitudes about food and practice healthy eating behaviors. *Bright Futures: Nutrition* can be used in a variety of community settings (eg, clinics, health and child care centers, hospitals, schools, colleges and universities). Community settings and events that provide a variety of healthy, affordable, and enjoyable foods can be instrumental in communicating positive nutrition messages.

Where We Go From Here

There are many opportunities to promote the nutrition status of infants, children, and adolescents. *Bright Futures: Nutrition* can be useful to health professionals, families, and communities as they strive to ensure the health and well-being of the current generation and of generations to come.

Nutrition Supervision

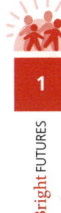

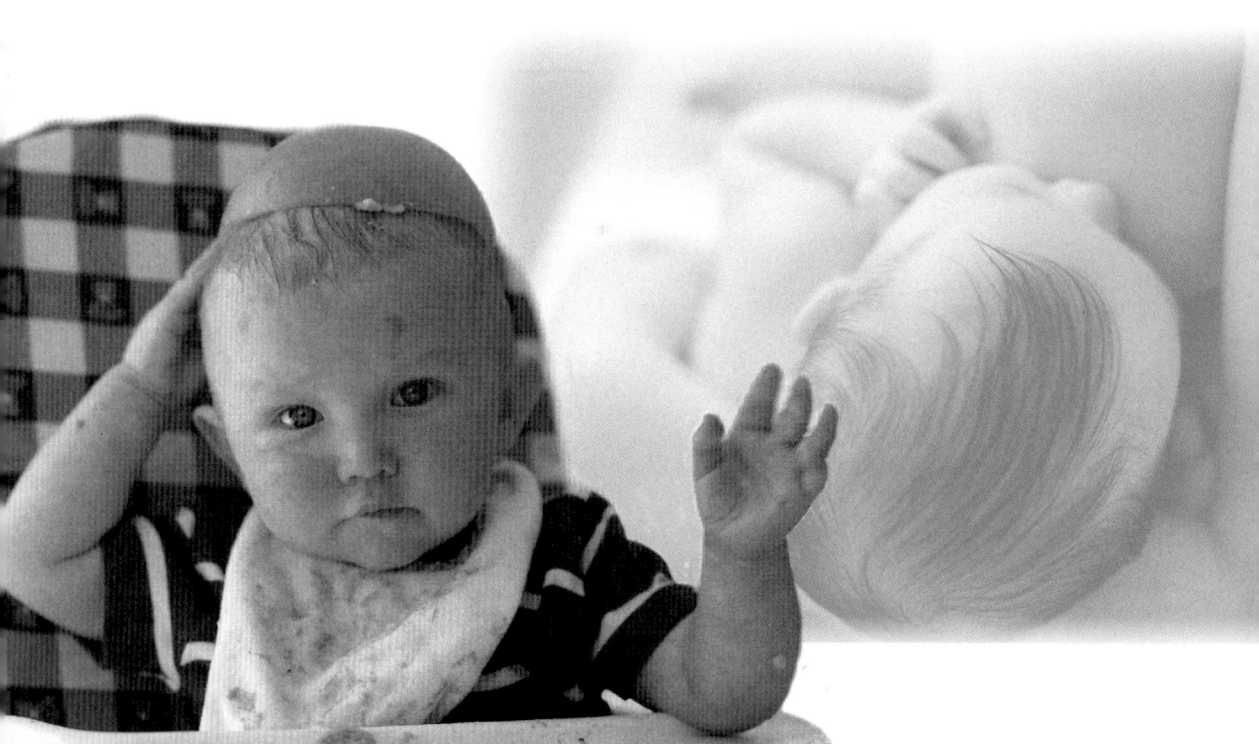

INFANCY

OVERVIEW

Infancy is divided into 3 stages. Physical growth, developmental achievements, nutrition needs, and feeding patterns vary significantly in each.

Early infancy (birth–age 6 months). The most rapid changes occur during this stage.

Middle infancy (ages 6–9 months). During this stage growth slows but is still rapid.

Late infancy (ages 9–12 months). During this stage growth slows, but infants' maturation and purposeful activity allow them to eat a wider variety of foods.

- Infants usually regain their birth weight by 7 days after birth, double their birth weight by age 4 to 6 months, and triple their birth weight by age 1.
- Infants usually increase their length by 50% in the first year, but the rate of increase slows during the second half of the year.
- Growth rates of exclusively breastfed infants and formula-fed infants differ. Breastfed infants grow more rapidly during the first half of the year but less rapidly during the second half.

- As infants grow, their ability to consume a greater volume and variety of food increases. Newborns need small, frequent feedings, whereas older infants are able to consume more volume at one time and require fewer feedings.
- Infants learn to chew and swallow, manipulate finger foods, drink from a cup, and ultimately feed themselves.
- In late infancy, infants' physical maturation, mastery of purposeful activity, and loss of newborn reflexes allow them to eat a wider variety foods, including foods with different textures, than they were able to consume during early and middle infancy.
- Close physical contact between the infant and a parent during feeding facilitates healthy social and emotional development.
- The amount and type of physical activity that an infant engages in change dramatically during infancy.
- At first, infants spend most of their time sleeping and eating. Over the next few months, infants slowly gain control over their movements. With increasing control comes more physical activity, including sitting up, rolling over, crawling, standing, and eventually walking.
- Development is an individual process. Infants typically acquire motor skills in the same order, but the speed at which they acquire them is different.

- The ways infants are held and handled, the toys they play with, and their environments all influence their physical activity and motor skills development.

COMMON NUTRITION CONCERNS

- Parents are often unsure whether to feed their infant breast milk or infant formula.
- After the new mother and the infant are discharged from the hospital, breastfeeding mothers may need breastfeeding guidance and referrals to lactation support services to provide follow-up care, phone consultation, follow-up visits, and help managing breastfeeding when the mother returns to work or when breastfeeding needs to be interrupted for any reason.
- Breastfeeding mothers of infants with special health care needs may need extra emotional support, instruction about special techniques for positioning, or special equipment to help overcome feeding problems.
- Infants with special health care needs may have feeding challenges that can be addressed as part of nutrition therapy in an early intervention program.
- Difficulties in early feeding evoke strong emotions in parents and can undermine parenting confidence and parents' sense of competency.

- Parents may need help in determining when to introduce solid foods into the infant's diet.

NUTRITION SUPERVISION

An infant's nutrition status should be evaluated during nutrition supervision visits or as part of health supervision visits. Health professionals can do the following:

- Begin nutrition supervision by selectively asking interview questions or by reviewing a questionnaire filled out by parents before the visit. Continue by conducting screening and assessment and providing anticipatory guidance.
- Recognize that interview questions, screening and assessment, and anticipatory guidance will vary from visit to visit and from infant to infant.

Nutrition pertaining to the entire developmental period is provided first in the pocket guide, followed by information on age-specific visits.

Interview Questions

- How do you think feeding is going for you and your baby? Do you have any questions about feeding your baby?
- How does your baby let you know when she is hungry? How do you know when she has had enough to eat?
- How often do you feed your baby?

- Does your baby receive anything else besides breast milk or infant formula?
- How do you feel about the way your baby is growing?
- Are you concerned about having enough money to buy food?
- What is the source of your drinking and cooking water? Do you use bottled or processed water?

Screening and Assessment

- Measure the infant's length, weight, and head circumference, and plot them on a standard growth chart. Deviation from expected growth patterns should be evaluated. This may be normal or may indicate a nutrition problem.
- Evaluate the appearance of the infant's skin, hair, teeth, gums, tongue, and eyes.
- Assess the infant for age-appropriate development.
- Observe the parent-infant interaction, and assess parents' and infants' responses to one another (affectionate, comfortable, distant, anxious).

Anticipatory Guidance

Discuss With Parents of All Infants

Feeding Practices

- Breast milk provides ideal nutrition and supports optimal growth and physical development. (Exclusive breastfeeding [only breast milk] is recommended for a minimum of 4 months, but preferably for 6 months.)
- Feeding their infant, until age 12 months, breast milk or iron-fortified infant formula and avoiding low-iron milk (cow's, goat's, soy), even in infant cereal.
- Feeding their infant until he is full.
- For younger infant (up to age 3 months), signs of hunger include putting the hand to the mouth, sucking, rooting, pre-cry facial grimaces, and fussing.
- For older infant (ages 4–6 months), signs of hunger include moving the head forward to reach the spoon and swiping food toward the mouth.
- Spitting up a little breast milk or formula at each feeding is normal.

Food Safety

- Following food safety practices for storage of expressed breast milk or open containers of ready-to-feed or concentrated formula.

- Dangers of warming expressed breast milk, formula, or food in containers or jars in the microwave.
- Warming bottles by holding them under hot running water or placing them in a bowl of hot water for a few minutes.
- Testing warmed fluids to make sure that they aren't too warm by sprinkling drops on wrist (the fluid should feel lukewarm; if too warm, cool down and test again).
- Avoiding foods that may cause choking (small or slippery foods, such as hard candy, whole grapes, hot dogs; dry and difficult-to-chew foods, such as popcorn, raw carrots, nuts; sticky or tough foods, such as peanut butter, large chunks of meat).
- Following food safety practices to reduce their infant's risk of food-borne illness.

(See Basics for Handling Food Safely.)

Supplements

- Giving breastfed and partially breastfed infants a vitamin D supplement beginning during the first few days of life. (Supplementation should continue unless the infant is weaned and is consuming at least 1 L per day or 1 qt per day of vitamin D–fortified formula or whole milk. Cow's milk should not be given to infants younger than 12 months.)
- Giving infants ingesting less than 1 L per day or 1 qt per day of vitamin D–fortified formula a vitamin D supplement beginning during the first few days of life.
- Giving breastfed infants vitamin B_{12} before age 6 months if the mother is vitamin B_{12} deficient (vegan [eats no animal products], is undernourished, does not take vitamin B_{12} supplements).

Oral Health

- Brushing their infant's teeth with a small, soft toothbrush and a smear of fluoridated toothpaste twice a day (after breakfast and before bed).
- Holding their infant while feeding, and never propping a bottle (using pillows or other objects to hold a bottle in their infant's mouth).
- Avoiding habits harmful to their infant's teeth (putting the infant to sleep with a bottle or sipper-type ["sippy"] cup or allowing frequent and prolonged bottle-feedings or use of a sippy cup containing beverages high in sugar).
- Maintaining personal oral health (visiting the dentist regularly, limiting foods and beverages high in sugar, and practicing good oral hygiene [brushing teeth twice a day with fluoridated toothpaste and flossing once a day]).

Physical Activity

- Discouraging television viewing and encouraging interactive activities (talking and reading together).

Discuss With Parents of Breastfed Infants

Feeding Practices

- Continuing breastfeeding for 12 months or as long as the mother and child wish to continue.
- Feeding their infant on demand stimulates the lactation process (the longer the infant sucks, the more breast milk the mother's body makes).
- Allowing their infant to finish feeding at one breast before offering the other breast (20–45 minutes per feeding provides adequate intake and allows the mother rest time between feedings).
- Feeding their infant when she is hungry, typically 10 to 12 times per day during the initial weeks of life, 8 to 12 times per day for the next several months, and 6 to 12 times per day thereafter.
- Feeding their infant more often during periods of rapid growth. (Frequent feedings help establish the milk supply and prevent the breasts from getting too full.)

Maternal Eating Behaviors

- Eating a variety of healthy foods helps the mother stay healthy and helps the infant grow.
- Drinking beverages such as milk or juice when thirsty and drinking a glass of water at each feeding.
- Limiting the consumption of beverages containing caffeine (coffee, tea, soft drinks) to 2 servings per day.
- Avoiding alcoholic beverages 2 hours before breastfeeding. (If the mother drinks alcoholic beverages, no more than 8 oz wine, 12 oz beer, or 2 oz hard liquor should be consumed per day [less for small women].)

Support

- Encouraging the father to help care for their infant (bringing the infant to the mother at breastfeeding time; cuddling the infant; helping with burping, diapering, and bathing).
- Mothers breastfeeding multiples require more food, additional nutrition counseling, and extra help at home.

Discuss With Parents of Formula-Fed Infants

Feeding Practices

- Holding their infant close when feeding, in a semi-upright position.
- Feeding their infant when he is hungry, typically every 3 to 4 hours (6–8 times in 24 hours) until complementary foods are added.
- Preparing and offering more formula as their infant's appetite increases.
- Offering their infant water on hot days between feedings (infants don't usually need water).
- Checking for causes if their infant is crying more than usual or seems hungry all the time (uncomfortable feeding position, formula prepared incorrectly, bottle nipple too firm or hole too big, unheeded hunger cues, distracting feeding environment).
- Not enlarging the hole in the bottle nipple to make infant formula come out faster.
- Seeking consultation with a health professional if their infant is not feeding enough.

Food Safety

- Preparing formula as instructed, and following sanitary procedures (washing hands before preparing formula; cleaning area where formula is prepared; cleaning and disinfecting reusable bottles, caps, and nipples before each use; washing and drying top of formula container before opening).
- Not adding cereal or other foods to infant formula.
- Discarding infant formula left in the bottle when their infant has finished eating; not reusing a bottle that has been started.
- Covering and refrigerating open containers of ready-to-feed or concentrated formula.
- Storing powdered formula at room temperature.

(See Basics for Handling Food Safely.)

PRENATAL

Interview Questions

For Pregnant Women

- What was your pre-pregnancy weight? How much weight did you gain in prior pregnancies? How much weight have you gained at this point?

- Are you taking or do you plan to take prenatal vitamins? Are you taking other vitamins or minerals?
- Have you used any special or traditional health remedies to improve your health since you have been pregnant?
- Do you drink alcohol or special teas or take any herbs? Is there anything that you were taking but stopped using when you learned that you were pregnant?
- Are you using any other drugs (legal or illegal) or supplements?
- What are your plans for feeding your baby? What have you heard about breastfeeding? Do you have questions about breastfeeding?
- Are you restricting any foods in your diet because of lack of appetite, food aversions, vegan or vegetarian diet, weight gain, food allergies and sensitivities, or any other reason?

For Women Planning to Breastfeed

- Do you have any worries about breastfeeding (your diet, privacy, having enough breast milk, changes in your body)? Have you had any breast surgery?
- Have you been to any classes that taught you how to nurse your baby?
- Do you know anyone who breastfeeds her baby? Did any of your family or friends breastfeed? Would you be able to get help from them as you are learning to breastfeed?

For Parents Planning to Formula-Feed

- What have you read or heard about different infant formulas (iron-fortified, soy, lactose-free)? Do you have any questions about formula-feeding?
- Are you worried about having enough money to buy infant formula?
- How do you plan to prepare the formula? What have you heard about formula safety?

Anticipatory Guidance

Discuss With Pregnant Women

- Obtain 600 dietary folate equivalents per day of food folate, folic acid, or a mixture of both to minimize the risk of giving birth to an infant with a neural tube defect.
- Consuming foods containing folate, such as fruits (oranges, strawberries, avocados), dark-green leafy vegetables (spinach, turnip greens), some other vegetables (asparagus, broccoli, brussels sprouts), and legumes (black, pinto, navy, and kidney beans).
- Consuming foods fortified with folic acid (grain products, most ready-to-eat breakfast cereals).
- Avoiding consumption of alcoholic beverages, because alcohol adversely affects fetal development.

Discuss With Women Planning to Breastfeed

- Herbal or traditional health remedies may be harmful to infants (many herbal teas contain ephedra and other substances that may be harmful).
- Giving breastfed and partially breastfed infants a vitamin D supplement beginning in the first few days of life. (Supplementation should continue unless the infant is weaned and is consuming at least 1 L per day or 1 qt per day of vitamin D–fortified formula or whole milk. Cow's milk should not be given to infants younger than 12 months.)

Discuss With Parents Planning to Formula-Feed

- Selecting infant formula and discussing any proposed changes in formula.
- Preparing infant formula (directions differ among powdered formulas), and heating and cleaning bottles and nipples.
- Feeding their infant on average 20 oz of formula in 24 hours (2 oz of infant formula every 2–3 hours at first and more formula if the infant seems hungry).
- Giving infants ingesting less than 1 L per day or 1 qt per day of vitamin D–fortified formula a vitamin D supplement beginning in the first few days of life.

NEWBORN

Interview Questions

For Parents of All Infants

- How often does your baby feed? How long does a feeding generally take?
- How does he behave during a feeding? Pulls away, arches back, is irritable or calm?
- How does your baby behave after feedings? Satisfied baby look, still rooting, anxious?
- Has your baby received any other fluids from a bottle?
- How many wet diapers and stools does your baby have each day?

For Parents of Breastfed Infants

- How often do you feed your baby? How do you know when he is hungry?
- How does your baby attach to your breast and suck? Do you hear him make swallowing sounds when you breastfeed?
- Have you had any problems with your breasts or nipples (tenderness, swelling, pain)?
- Are you restricting any foods in your diet?

- What vitamin or mineral supplements do you take or plan to take? Is your baby receiving vitamin D supplements?
- Do you drink wine, beer, or other alcoholic beverages? Do you drink any special teas or take any herbs?
- Do you use any drugs (prescription, over the counter, street drugs)?

For Parents of Formula-Fed Infants

- What formula are you planning to use? Is the formula iron-fortified?
- How often do you feed your baby? How much does she take at a feeding?
- What questions do you have about infant formula (brands, cost, preparation, amount)?
- How do you store the infant formula after you make it?
- How do you clean bottles, nipples, and other equipment?
- What do you do with the formula in the bottle after your baby has finished feeding?
- How does your baby like to be held when you feed her?
- Are you worried about having enough money to buy infant formula?

Screening and Assessment

- Perform metabolic screening as indicated by the state.
- Assess administration of vitamin K.

Anticipatory Guidance

Discuss With Parents of All Infants

- Signs of hunger include putting the hand to the mouth, sucking, rooting, pre-cry facial grimaces, and fussing (crying is a late sign hunger).
- Waking their infant for feeding if the infant sleeps more than 4 hours.
- Helping their infant focus on feeding by rocking, patting, stroking, or swaddling the infant or feeding in a room with fewer distractions (lights, noise).

Discuss With Parents of Breastfed Infants

- Feeding their infant immediately after birth, preferably in the delivery room.
- Feeding their infant when she is hungry, usually every 2 to 3 hours, about 8 to 12 feedings in 24 hours.
- Their infant is getting enough milk if there are 6 to 8 wet diapers and 3 or 4 stools in 24 hours and the infant is gaining weight as expected.
- Avoiding artificial nipples (pacifiers, bottles) and supplements (unless medically indicated) until breastfeeding is well established; this occurs at around age 4 to 6 weeks. (Some infants never use pacifiers or bottles.)

- Waiting until breastfeeding is well established before introducing infant formula (for mothers combining breastfeeding and formula-feeding).

Discuss With Parents of Formula-Fed Infants

- Feeding their infant on average 20 oz of formula in 24 hours (2 oz of infant formula every 2–3 hours at first and more formula if the infant seems hungry).

3 TO 5 DAYS

Interview Questions

For Parents of All Infants

- How are you feeding your baby?
- How often does your baby feed? How long does it generally take for a feeding?
- How does your baby like to be held when you feed him?
- Are you comfortable that your baby is getting enough to eat?
- How does he behave during a feeding? Pulls away, arches back, is irritable, or calm?
- How does your baby behave after feedings? Satisfied baby look, still rooting, anxious?
- Has he received any other fluids from a bottle?

- How many wet diapers and stools does he have each day?
- What is the longest time he has slept at one time?

For Parents of Breastfed Infants

- How is breastfeeding going for you and your baby?
- Is your baby receiving a vitamin D supplement?
- Does your baby suck well? Does she latch on well and breastfeed in a rhythm?
- Do you feel a good "let-down" or "milk-ejection" reflex (tingling sensation and a strong surge of milk)?
- Have you noticed changes in your milk?
- How often does your baby feed? How long do feedings last?

For Parents of Formula-Fed Infants

- What formula are you feeding your baby? Is it iron-fortified?
- How are you preparing the formula?
- How often do you feed your baby? How much does he take at a feeding?
- How do you hold your baby while feeding? How do you hold the bottle?
- What questions do you have about infant formula (brands, cost, preparation, amount)?
- What questions do you have about preparing formula and storing it safely?

- Are you worried about having enough money to buy infant formula?

Screening and Assessment

- Perform metabolic screening as indicated by the state.
- Assess the infant for milk intake, hydration, jaundice, and age-appropriate elimination patterns.
- If possible, observe the mother breastfeeding or either parent bottle-feeding the infant. Assess how comfortable the parent seems with feeding the infant, eye contact between the parent and the infant, the parent's interaction with the infant, the parent's and the infant's responses to distractions in the environment, and the infant's ability to suck.

Anticipatory Guidance

Discuss With Parents of All Infants

- Signs of hunger include infant putting the hand in the mouth, sucking, rooting, pre-cry facial grimaces, and fussing (crying is a late sign hunger).
- Waking their infant for feeding if the infant sleeps for more than 4 hours.

- Helping their infant focus on feeding by rocking, patting, stroking, or swaddling the infant or feeding in a room with fewer distractions (lights, noise).

Discuss With Parents of Breastfed Infants

- Their infant settling into typical breastfeeding routine of every 2 to 3 hours in the daytime and every 3 hours at night, with 4- to 5-hour stretches between feedings; total of 10 to 12 feedings in 24 hours.
- After the mother's milk comes in, infants should have about 6 to 8 wet diapers in 24 hours. (Infants may have stools [typically loose] after every feeding or as infrequently as every several days.)
- Avoiding artificial nipples (pacifiers, bottles) and supplements (unless medically indicated) until breastfeeding is well established; this occurs around age 4 to 6 weeks. (Some infants never use pacifiers or bottles.)

Discuss With Parents of Formula-Fed Infants

- Feeding their infant on average 20 oz of formula in 24 hours (2 oz of formula every 2–3 hours at first and more formula if the infant seems hungry).

BY 1 MONTH

Interview Questions

For Parents of All Infants

- How often are you feeding your baby during the day? During the night?
- How do you know if your baby is hungry? How do you know if your baby has had enough food?
- Have there been times when she seemed to be growing very fast and seemed to want to eat all the time? What did you do?
- How easily does your baby burp during or after a feeding?
- How many wet diapers and stools does your baby have each day?
- What is the longest time your baby has slept?
- Are you giving your baby any supplements, herbs, or vitamins?

For Parents of Breastfed Infants

- Are you breastfeeding exclusively? If not, what else are you feeding your baby?
- How often do you feed your baby? How long do you feed him each time?
- Are you breastfeeding more often or for longer periods?
- How can you tell if your baby is satisfied at the breast?
- Are you planning to return to work or school? If so, are you pumping your breast milk? How do you store it? How long do you keep it?

For Parents of Formula-Fed Infants

- Do you ever prop a bottle to feed your baby or put her to bed with a bottle?
- What formula do you use? Is the formula iron-fortified?
- How often does your baby feed? How much does she take at a feeding?
- How long does it take to feed your baby?
- Have you given your baby anything other than infant formula?
- What concerns do you have about infant formula (cost, preparation, nutrient content)?
- Are you worried about having enough money to buy infant formula?

Screening and Assessment

- If possible, observe the mother breastfeeding or either parent bottle-feeding the infant. Assess how comfortable the parent seems with feeding the infant, eye contact between the parent and the infant, the parent's interaction with the infant, the parent's and the infant's responses to distractions in the environment, and the infant's ability to suck.
- For breastfed and partially breastfed infants, determine whether the infant is receiving vitamin D supplementation.

Anticipatory Guidance

Discuss With Parents of All Infants

- Their infant's increasing appetite during growth spurts, between ages 6 and 8 weeks.
- Forgoing foods other than breast milk or infant formula until their infant is developmentally ready (at about age 4–6 months, when the sucking reflex changes to allow coordinated swallowing and the infant is sitting with support and has good head and neck control).

- Helping their infant focus on feeding by rocking, patting, stroking, or swaddling the infant or feeding in a room with fewer distractions (lights, noise).
- Indications of colic (crying inconsolably for several hours and passing a lot of gas). (If the mother is breastfeeding, recommend short, frequent feedings.)

Discuss With Parents of Breastfed Infants

- Their infant is getting enough milk if there are 6 to 8 wet diapers and 3 or 4 stools in 24 hours and the infant is gaining weight as expected.
- When appropriate, introducing a bottle by someone other than the mother when their infant is neither extremely hungry nor full and allowing the infant to explore the bottle's nipple and put it in his mouth.

Discuss With Parents of Formula-Fed Infants

- Feeding their infant on average 24 to 27 oz of formula, but the infant may consume 20 to 31 oz of formula in 24 hours. (Infant needs to feed every 3–4 hours.)

15

2 MONTHS

Interview Questions

For Parents of All Infants

- Tell me about all the foods you are offering your baby.
- Have there been times when he seemed to be growing very fast and seemed to want to eat all the time? What did you do?

For Parents of Breastfed Infants

- How often do you feed your baby? How long do you feed her each time?
- Does it seem like your baby is breastfeeding more often or for longer periods?
- Does your baby receive other foods or fluids besides breast milk?
- Are you planning to return to work or school? If so, will you pump your breast milk?
- Does your school or workplace have a place where you can pump your milk in privacy? How will you store your milk? How long will you keep it?

For Parents of Formula-Fed Infants

- How often does your baby feed? How much does he drink at a feeding?
- About how long does a feeding last? Have you offered him anything other than formula?
- Do you ever prop a bottle to feed or put your baby to bed with a bottle?
- Are you worried about having enough money to buy infant formula?

Screening and Assessment

- Observe parent/infant interaction (gazing, talking, smiling, holding, cuddling, comforting).
- If possible, observe the mother breastfeeding or either parent bottle-feeding the infant. Assess how comfortable the parent seems with feeding the infant, eye contact between parent and infant, the parent's interaction with the infant, the parent's and the infant's responses to distractions in the environment, and the infant's ability to suck.
- For breastfed infants, determine whether the infant is receiving vitamin D supplementation.

Discuss With Parents of All Infants

- Growing infants are more easily distracted during feeding and need gentle, repetitive stimulation (rocking, patting, stroking) or feeding in a room with fewer distractions (lights, noise, other people).
- Indications of colic (crying inconsolably for several hours and passing a lot of gas). (If the mother is breastfeeding, recommend short, frequent feedings.)
- Forgoing foods other than breast milk or infant formula until their infant is developmentally ready (at about age 4–6 months, when the sucking reflex changes to allow coordinated swallowing and the infant is sitting with support and has good head and neck control).
- Adding cereal to their infant's diet will not help the infant sleep through the night.
- Playing with their infant (encouraging the infant to follow objects with his eyes) to stimulate the nervous system and help develop head and neck control and motor skills.
- Encouraging "tummy time" to promote head control and gross motor development.

Discuss With Parents of Breastfed Infants

- Breastfeeding their infant 8 to 12 times in 24 hours, and feeding more frequently during growth spurts.
- By age 3 months, feeding their infant every 2 to 3 hours, but they may have one longer stretch of 4 to 5 hours at night between feedings.
- Stools may be as infrequent as once every 3 days.

Discuss With Parents of Formula-Fed Infants

- Feeding their infant on average 26 to 28 oz of formula, but the infant may consume up to 32 oz of formula in 24 hours (infants feed every 3–4 hours, with one longer stretch at night of up to 5 or 6 hours between feedings).

4 MONTHS

Interview Questions

For Parents of All Infants

- Tell me about what you are feeding your baby. How often are you feeding her?
- Are you feeding your baby any foods besides breast milk or formula?
- Have you thought about when you will begin to give your baby solids?

- Does your baby seem interested in your food?
- Have you offered her foods from the family meal? If so, which ones?
- In addition to feeding her at home, where else is she fed (child care, relative's home)?

For Parents of Breastfed Infants

- In what ways is breastfeeding different now from when you were last here?
- Is your baby breastfeeding more often or for longer periods?
- How can you tell whether he is satisfied at the breast?
- Has he received breast milk or other fluids from a bottle?
- Are you giving your baby any supplements (vitamin D, iron)?
- Are you planning to return to work or school? If so, are you pumping your breast milk? How are you storing pumped breast milk? How long do you keep it?

For Parents of Formula-Fed Infants

- What formula are you using? Is the formula iron-fortified?
- How often does your baby feed? How much at a feeding? How much in 24 hours?
- Has your baby begun to put her hands around the bottle?
- Have you offered your baby anything other than infant formula?

- Are you worried about having enough money to buy infant formula?

Screening and Assessment

- For breastfed infants, determine whether the infant is receiving vitamin D supplementation and whether the infant is receiving iron-rich foods or iron supplementation.

Anticipatory Guidance

Discuss With Parents of All Infants

- Responding to their infant's feeding cues indicating hunger (moving the head forward to reach the bottle or spoon) or fullness (leaning back and turning away from food).
- Forgoing foods other than breast milk or infant formula until the infant is developmentally ready (at about age 4–6 months, when the sucking reflex changes to allow coordinated swallowing and the infant is sitting with support and has good head and neck control).
- Introducing one single-ingredient food at a time, and observing the infant for 3 to 5 days for possible allergic reactions.

- Introducing iron-fortified, single-grain infant rice cereal as the first supplemental food because it is least likely to cause an allergic reaction.
- Introducing a variety of pureed or soft meats, fruits, and vegetables after cereals. (The gradual introduction of a variety of foods, flavors, and textures contributes to a balanced diet and helps promote healthy eating behaviors.)

Discuss With Parents of Breastfed Infants

- A demand for more frequent breastfeeding is usually related to their infant's growth spurt. If an increased demand continues for a few days; is not affected by increased breastfeeding; and is unrelated to illness, teething, or changes in routine, it may be a sign that the infant is ready for solid foods.
- Providing a vitamin D supplement (400 IU/day).
- Providing an iron supplement (1 mg/kg of body weight/day) if the infant does not consume sufficient iron-rich foods.

Discuss With Parents of Formula-Fed Infants

- Feeding their infant on average 30 to 32 oz of formula, but the infant may consume up to 26 to 36 oz of formula in 24 hours.

- Vitamin supplements are not needed if their infant is consuming an adequate amount of iron-fortified infant formula appropriate for growth.

6 MONTHS

Interview Questions

For Parents of All Infants

- What are you feeding your baby at this time?
- Have you thought about when you will begin to give your baby solids?
- How are you planning to introduce solid foods, such as cereal, fruits, vegetables, meats, and other foods?
- Has he eaten any foods from the family meal? If so, which ones?
- What types of fluids is your baby getting in a bottle or cup?

For Parents of Breastfed Infants

- How often are you breastfeeding your baby? For how long on each breast?
- Does it seem like your baby is breastfeeding more often or for longer periods?
- What are your plans for continuing to breastfeed?

- Has your baby received breast milk or other fluids from a bottle or cup?
- Is your baby receiving vitamin D supplements?
- Is your baby receiving an iron supplement and/or iron-rich foods?

For Parents of Formula-Fed Infants

- How is formula-feeding going? What formula are you using now?
- How often does your baby feed in 24 hours, and how much does she take at a feeding? Day feedings versus night feedings?

Screening and Assessment

- Assess eating behaviors to determine the infant's risk for dental caries (tooth decay). Determine whether the infant has had a dental visit.
- For breastfed infants, determine whether the infant is receiving vitamin D supplementation, and assess the need for iron supplementation.

Anticipatory Guidance

Discuss With Parents of All Infants

- Introducing solid foods when their infant is developmentally ready (at about age 4–6 months, when the sucking reflex changes to allow coordinated swallowing and the infant is sitting with support and has good head and neck control).
- Introducing one single-ingredient food at a time, and observing their infant for 3 to 5 days for possible allergic reactions.
- Introducing iron-fortified, single-grain infant rice cereal as the first supplemental food, because it is least likely to cause an allergic reaction.
- Introducing a variety of pureed or soft meats, fruits, and vegetables after cereals.
- Not forcing their infant to eat a new food if the infant does not like it. (It may take 10–15 attempts before an infant accepts a particular food.)
- Serving only 100% fruit juice in a cup as part of a meal or snack, and limiting juice to 4 to 6 oz per day.
- Placing their infant in a high chair (using a safety belt) to sit with the family during mealtime.

- Talking with their infant during feedings. (As infants develop, they increasingly respond to social interaction.)
- Infants benefit from playing with toys for stacking, shaking, pushing, or dropping and from playing with others.

Discuss With Parents of Breastfed Infants
- Encouraging the mother to breastfeed for the first year of the infant's life.
- Providing a vitamin D supplement (400 IU/day).
- Providing an iron supplement (1 mg/kg of body weight/day) if the infant does not consume sufficient iron-rich foods.

Discuss With Parents of Formula-Fed Infants
- Feeding their infant when the infant is hungry, usually 5 to 6 times in 24 hours.
- Vitamin supplements are not needed if the infant is consuming an adequate amount of iron-fortified infant formula appropriate for growth.

9 MONTHS

Interview Questions

For Parents of All Infants
- How has feeding been going? What questions or concerns do you have?
- Who feeds your baby?
- When does your baby have something to eat or drink? How much does he eat or drink at a time?
- Is your baby drinking less breast milk or infant formula?
- Is your baby interested in feeding himself? What is he feeding himself?
- What does your baby eat with his fingers? Has he used a cup?
- Is your baby interested in the food you eat?
- What does your baby do when he has had enough to eat?
- Do you know what your baby eats when he is away from home (at child care)?

For Parents of Breastfed Infants
- What are your plans for continuing to breastfeed? How often does your baby breastfeed? How long do you feed her each time?
- How is your milk supply?

- Is your baby receiving vitamin D supplementation?
- Has your baby had infant formula or cow's, goat's, or soy milk?
- Is your baby receiving an iron supplement and/or iron-rich foods?

For Parents of Formula-Fed Infants

- What formula are you using now?
- How often does your baby feed in 24 hours? How much does he take at a feeding? Day feedings versus night feedings?
- How are you preparing infant formula for your baby?
- What kind of water is used to prepare the formula? Does the water contain fluoride?
- Do you have any questions about weaning your baby from the bottle?
- Are you worried about having enough money to buy infant formula?

Screening and Assessment

Iron-Deficiency Anemia

Guidelines from the American Academy of Pediatrics (AAP) and the Centers for Disease Control and Prevention (CDC):

- Screen infants at about age 12 months. (AAP)
- Screen infants at high risk or those with known risk factors at ages 9 to 12 months and again 6 months later (ages 15–18 months). (CDC)
  - Infants considered at high risk for iron-deficiency anemia include
    - ► Infants from families with low incomes
    - ► Infants who are eligible for Special Supplemental Nutrition Program for Women, Infants, and Children (WIC)
    - ► Infants who are migrants or recently arrived refugees
    - ► Infants and children who are Mexican American
  - Infants who have known risk factors for iron-deficiency anemia include
    - ► Infants born preterm or with low birth weight
    - ► Infants fed non–iron-fortified infant formula for more than 2 months
    - ► Infants fed cow's milk before age 12 months
    - ► Infants who are breastfed and who do not receive adequate iron from supplemental foods after age 4 months

Lead Exposure

- Screen the infant for lead exposure.

Oral Health

■ Assess eating behaviors to determine the infant's risk for dental caries (tooth decay). Determine whether the infant has had a dental visit.

Vitamin D and Iron

■ For breastfed infants, determine whether the infant is receiving vitamin D supplementation, and assess the need for iron supplementation.

Anticipatory Guidance

Discuss With Parents of All Infants

■ Gradually introducing their infant to solid textures to decrease the risk of feeding problems, such as rejecting certain textures, refusing to chew, or vomiting. (It may take 10–15 attempts before an infant accepts a particular food.)

■ Understanding that infants will become more interested in food their parents eat and less interested in breastfeeding or bottle-feeding. Nevertheless, infants should receive breast milk, infant formula, or both through the first year of life.

■ Offering soft, moist foods as their infant gradually moves from gumming to chewing foods.

■ Offering small pieces of soft foods as their infant gains more control over picking up and holding food.

■ Placing their infant in a high chair (using a safety belt) to sit with the family during mealtime.

■ Serving only 100% fruit juice in a cup as part of a meal or snack, and limiting juice to 4 to 6 oz per day.

■ Avoiding feeding their infant sweetened beverages, such as sodas and fruit drinks.

■ Providing their infant snacks midmorning, in the afternoon, and in the evening. (Most 9-month-olds are on the same eating schedule as the family: breakfast, lunch, and dinner.)

Discuss With Parents of Breastfed Infants

■ Encouraging the mother to breastfeed for the first year of the infant's life.

■ Providing vitamin D supplement (400 IU/day).

■ Providing an iron supplement (1 mg/kg of body weight/day) if the infant does not consume sufficient iron-rich foods.

Discuss With Parents of Formula-Fed Infants

- Feeding the infant when the infant is hungry, usually 5 to 6 times in 24 hours.
- Vitamin supplements are not needed if the infant is consuming an adequate amount of iron-fortified infant formula appropriate for growth.

EARLY CHILDHOOD

OVERVIEW

Early childhood is a period during which physical, cognitive, social, and emotional development are tightly linked. The period is divided into 2 stages.

Toddler (ages 1–2). Toddlers are characterized by a growing sense of independence and sometimes by struggles over food and refusing to eat certain foods. They are developing fine motor skills, so eating is often messy.

Young child (ages 3–4). Young children are increasingly competent at self-feeding, but they still prefer eating with their hands rather than using utensils. They are becoming more interested in trying new foods and participating in family meals.

- Children quadruple their birth weight by age 2.
- Between ages 2 and 5, children gain an average of 4.5 to 6.5 lbs and grow 2.5 to 3.5 inches per year.
- As growth rates decline during early childhood, children's appetites decrease, and the amount of food they consume may become unpredictable.
- As toddlers' eating skills develop, they progress from eating soft pieces of food to eating foods with more texture.
- Toddlers tend to be leery of new foods and may refuse to eat them. They need to look at the new foods and touch, smell, and taste them many times before they accept them.
- Toddlers are unpredictable. They may like certain foods one day and dislike them the next. They may eat a lot one day and very little the next.
- By age 3 or 4, children are able to use their fingers to push food onto a spoon, pick up food with a fork, and drink from a cup.
- Most young children become more curious about food than they were as toddlers, although they still may be reluctant to try new foods.
- As young children grow, they become less impulsive and can follow instructions. They can serve themselves from bowls and plates and pass food to others. Young children are more comfortable eating in unfamiliar places than they were as toddlers.
- Early childhood is a key time for promoting the development of motor skills and good habits for physical activity that will last a lifetime.
- Parents need to plan activities so that children can master control of their large muscles but still have time to just play.
- Physical activities (running, jumping, climbing, throwing, catching) and simple games (Simon Says, chase, tag) are appropriate during early childhood.

- Young children are not ready for organized, competitive sports, which require visual acuity, control, cooperation, and balance.
- Being physically active helps ensure that children maintain a healthy weight.

COMMON NUTRITION CONCERNS

- Obesity prevalence has risen from 5% to more than 12% among children ages 2 to 5.
- Children who are obese often remain obese into adulthood, and higher degrees of excess weight are associated with increasing risk of persistent obesity. Obesity is associated with many chronic health conditions, including diabetes mellitus, hypertension, dyslipidemia, and cardiovascular disease.
- Iron deficiency and iron-deficiency anemia are common in children, especially children from families with low incomes. Iron-deficiency anemia may have adverse effects on growth and development.
- Children with special health care needs may have nutrition concerns, including poor growth, poor eating skills, inadequate or excessive food intake, developmental delays, elimination problems, and metabolic disorders.

(See Key Indicators of Nutrition Risk for Children and Adolescents.)

NUTRITION SUPERVISION

A child's nutrition status should be evaluated during nutrition supervision visits or as part of health supervision visits. Health professionals can do the following:

- Begin nutrition supervision by selectively asking interview questions or by reviewing a questionnaire filled out by parents before the visit. Continue by conducting screening and assessment and providing anticipatory guidance.
- Recognize that interview questions, screening and assessment, and anticipatory guidance will vary from visit to visit and from child to child.

Nutrition pertaining to the entire developmental period is provided first in the pocket guide, followed by information on age-specific visits.

Interview Questions

- What concerns do you have about your child's eating behaviors or growth?
- How does your child let you know when she is hungry and when she is full?

- Describe what your child does during mealtimes. What do you do?
- What do you do if your child doesn't like a particular food?
- Do you have equipment for feeding your child (cups, forks and spoons, a high chair, a booster seat)?
- Do you have any concerns about the food served to her when she is away from home?
- Are you concerned about having enough money to buy food?

Screening and Assessment

Growth and Development

- Measure the child's length or height and the child's weight, and plot it on a standard growth chart. Deviation from expected growth patterns should be evaluated. This may be normal or may indicate a nutrition problem.
- Determine the child's nutrition status and overall health using body mass index (BMI). Calculate the child's BMI by dividing weight by square of height (kg/m^2), or use a BMI wheel or calculator. Plot the child's BMI and age on a BMI-for-age growth chart to determine BMI percentile.
- Evaluate the appearance of the child's skin, hair, teeth, gums, tongue, and eyes.

Iron-Deficiency Anemia

Guidelines from the American Academy of Pediatrics (AAP) and the Centers for Disease Control and Prevention (CDC):

Children Ages 12 to 18 Months

- Screen children at about age 12 months and about age 18 months. (AAP)
- Screen children at high risk or those with known risk factors at ages 9 to 12 months and again 6 months later (ages 15–18 months). (CDC)
  - Children considered to be at high risk for iron-deficiency anemia include
    - ▸ Children from families with low incomes
    - ▸ Children who are eligible for the Special Supplemental Nutrition Program for Women, Infants, and Children (WIC)
    - ▸ Children who are migrants or recently arrived refugees
    - ▸ Children who are Mexican American

- Children who have known risk factors for iron-deficiency anemia include
  - ▸ Children born preterm or with low birth weight
  - ▸ Children fed non–iron-fortified infant formula for more than 2 months
  - ▸ Children fed cow's milk before age 12 months
  - ▸ Children who are breastfed and do not receive adequate iron from supplemental foods after age 4 months
  - ▸ Children who consume more than 24 oz of cow's milk per day
  - ▸ Children with special health care needs who use medications that interfere with iron absorption (eg, antacids, calcium, phosphorus, magnesium) or those with chronic infection; inflammatory disorders; restricted diets; or extensive blood loss from a wound, an accident, or surgery.

Children Ages 2 to 5

- Screen children annually if the following risk factors are present (AAP):
  - Special health care needs
  - Diet low in iron
  - Vegetarian diet
  - Low socioeconomic status
  - Limited access to food
- Screen children annually if the following risk factors are present (CDC):
  - Diet low in iron
  - Limited access to food because of poverty or neglect
  - Special health care needs
  - Low income
  - Eligible for WIC
  - Migrant or recently arrived refugee

Oral Health

- Determine whether the child has regular dental visits.
- Assess eating behaviors (frequency of consuming foods and beverages high in sugar) to determine the child's risk for dental caries (tooth decay).

Physical Activity

- Determine how much physical activity the child engages in weekly.
- Determine how much time the child spends watching television and engaging in other media activities (computer, video games). Determine whether the child watches television during mealtimes.

Discuss With Parents

Parent-Child Feeding Relationship

- Purchasing and preparing nutritious food.
- Offering developmentally appropriate, healthy meals and snacks at scheduled times in a pleasant environment.
- Helping their child develop eating and self-serving skills (progressing from using hands for eating to using utensils).
- Helping their child learn to self-regulate food intake by responding to internal cues of hunger and fullness.
- Allowing their child to decide whether to eat and how much.

Meals and Snacks

- Offering healthy food choices at meals and snacks served at about the same time each day.
- Offering nutritious foods (whole-grain crackers, milk and milk products, fruits, vegetables, meat or poultry) as snacks because children often eat small amounts of food at one time.
- Sharing meals and snacks with their child. (Children eat better when an adult is nearby.)
- Being positive role models by eating new foods.

- Making family mealtimes a priority, and getting rid of distractions (television).
- Being patient and understanding as their child learns to feed or serve herself.
- Offering small portions (1 or 2 tablespoons) of new foods.
- Not using foods to reward, bribe, or punish their child or to calm, comfort, or entertain her.
- Offering dessert (custard, pudding, fruits, yogurt) as part of a meal.

Eating

- Weaning their child from the bottle by age 12 to 14 months.
- Modifying foods to make them easier for their child to eat.
- Helping children ages 2 to 5 gradually decrease their fat intake.
- Serving children ages 1 to 2 whole milk (serving reduced-fat [2%] milk if obesity is of concern or if there is a family history of obesity, dyslipidemia, or cardiovascular disease).
- Serving children older than age 2 low-fat (1%) or fat-free (skim) milk.
- Serving children ages 2 and older 2 servings of milk (two 8-oz cups) per day.

- Serving children grain products, especially whole grains; fruits; vegetables; milk and milk products; and beans, lean meat, poultry, fish, and other protein-rich foods.
- Providing children ages 2 to 3 with the same number of servings as children ages 4 and older, but with smaller portions (about two-thirds of a serving).
- Serving children ages 4 and older portion sizes similar to those eaten by older family members (½ cup of fruits or vegetables; ¾ cup of 100% fruit juice; 1 slice of whole-grain bread; 2–3 oz of cooked lean meat, poultry, or fish).
- Providing a vitamin D supplement of 400 IU per day for children who do not obtain 400 IU per day of vitamin D through vitamin D–fortified milk (100 IU per 8-oz serving) and vitamin D–fortified foods (fortified cereals, eggs [yolks]).
- Serving 100% fruit juice in a cup; limiting consumption to 4 to 6 oz per day.
- Reducing risk of dental caries (tooth decay), minor infections, and loose stools and diarrhea by not allowing their child to drink unlimited amounts of fruit juices or sweetened beverages (fruit drinks, soft drinks).
- Maintaining their child's appetite for healthy foods by limiting foods (candy, cookies) and beverages (fruit drinks, soft drinks) high in sugar.
- Encouraging their child to drink water throughout day.

Food Safety

- Following food safety practices to reduce their child's risk of food-borne illnesses.
- Having their child sit in a high chair or booster seat during feeding.
- Using techniques for positioning or special equipment or modifying utensils for feeding children with special health care needs.
- Following precautions to prevent their child from choking.
  - Staying with their child while eating.
  - Having their child sit while eating.
  - Not allowing their child to eat in the car.
  - Keeping mealtimes and snack times calm.
  - Avoiding foods that may cause their toddler to choke (hard candy, mini-marshmallows, popcorn, pretzels, chips, spoonfuls of peanut butter, nuts, seeds, large chunks of meat, hot dogs, raw carrots, raisins and other dried fruits, whole grapes).
- Modifying foods for their young child to make them safer (cutting hot dogs in quarters lengthwise and then into small pieces, cutting whole grapes in half lengthwise, chopping nuts finely, chopping raw carrots finely or into thin strips, spreading peanut butter thinly on crackers or bread).

(See Basics for Handling Food Safely.)

Teaching Children About Food

- Offering a variety of healthy foods.
- Offering foods from other cultures.
- Teaching child how foods are grown (planting a vegetable garden) and where foods come from (visiting a dairy farm).
- Reading books and singing songs about foods.
- Involving their child in food shopping and preparation.

Oral Health

- For children ages 1 to 2, brushing the child's teeth with a small, soft toothbrush and a smear of fluoridated toothpaste twice a day (after breakfast and before bed).
- For children ages 2 and older, brushing the child's teeth with a small, soft toothbrush and a pea-sized amount of fluoridated toothpaste twice a day (after breakfast and before bed).
- Toothbrushing requires good fine motor control, and young children cannot clean their teeth without help. (After children acquire fine motor skills [ability to tie their shoelaces], typically by age 7 or 8, they can brush their teeth effectively.)
- Drinking water when thirsty.

- Using community fluoridated water as a safe, effective was to reduce dental caries. (If bottled water is preferred, recommend a brand with fluoride added at a concentration of approximately 0.8–1.0 mg/L [ppm].)
- Limiting foods (candy, cookies) and beverages (juice, juice drinks, soft drinks) high in sugar.

Physical Activity

- Promoting both structured (following the leader) and free (child moves in any way he likes) play.
- Playing with their child and being physically active. (Parents' involvement and enthusiasm in physical activity have a positive impact on their child's play experiences.)
- Planning family activities each week to encourage being physically active.
- Letting their child decide which physical activities the family will do (walking, hiking, playing tag).
- Taking part in community projects as a family (neighborhood cleanup days, community gardens, food drives).
- Encouraging interactive activities (playing, singing, and reading together).
- Limiting their child's total entertainment media time (watching television, playing computer or video games) to no more than 1 to 2 hours of quality programming a day.

1 YEAR

Interview Questions

- Are you breastfeeding your child?
- What type of infant formula or milk do you feed him?
- Does your child drink from a cup? Does he drink from a bottle now and then? If so, what are your plans for weaning him from the bottle?
- What textures of food does your child eat? Does he eat pieces of soft food?
- Does he eat with the family?

Screening and Assessment

- Screen the child for lead exposure.
- Evaluate the child's progress in developing eating skills. Make sure the child
  - Can bite off small pieces of food
  - Can put food in the mouth
  - Has an adequate gag reflex
  - Can retain food in the mouth (doesn't immediately swallow)
  - Can chew food using an up-and-down or rotary motion
  - Can use a pincer grasp to pick up small pieces of food
  - Can drink from a cup

- Evaluate the child's interest in active play (bouncing, crawling, climbing).

Anticipatory Guidance

Discuss With Parents

- Giving their child opportunities to develop eating skills (chewing, swallowing) by offering a variety of healthy foods and feeding at a family table.
- Serving beverages in a cup. (Children may need help drinking from a cup.)
- Offering their child food every 2 to 3 hours. (Children's capacity to eat at any one time is limited.)
- Handling their child's limit-testing behaviors (asking for certain foods and throwing tantrums when refused).
- Imposing limits on their child's unacceptable mealtime behaviors without controlling the amount or types of foods the child eats.
- Discouraging television viewing and encouraging interactive activities (talking, playing, singing, and reading together).

15 MONTHS

Interview Questions

- Are you breastfeeding your child? Are you giving her bottles? Milk in a cup? What kind of milk does she drink? How much?
- How much fruit juice or how many sweetened drinks (fruit drinks, soft drinks) does your child drink? Is the juice 100% fruit juice? When does she drink them?
- Which foods does your child like to eat? Are there any foods she doesn't like?
- Describe your child's mealtimes. Does she eat with the family?
- Does she ask for food between meals and snacks? If so, how do you handle this?
- Does your child throw tantrums over food? If so, how do you handle them?
- What kinds of physical activities does your child enjoy?
- What concerns do you have about your child's weight?

Screening and Assessment

- Evaluate the child's progress in developing large motor skills. Children should be actively playing with a parent daily.

Anticipatory Guidance

Discuss With Parents

- Offering their child food every 2 to 3 hours. (Children's capacity to eat at any one time is limited.)
- Giving their child opportunities to develop eating skills (chewing, swallowing) by offering a variety of foods and eating at a family table.
- Offering age-appropriate foods (cut food into small pieces) and continuing to monitor the size of foods. (Chewing and swallowing functions are not completely developed until about age 8.)
- Making eating easier for their child by using spoons, cups, and dishes with steep sides (bowls).
- Being patient as their child's skill at eating a variety of foods increases.
- Providing a relaxed atmosphere during meals and snacks. (Children should not be rushed, because trying new foods takes time.)
- Discouraging television viewing and encouraging interactive activities (talking, playing, singing, and reading together).

18 MONTHS

Interview Questions

- Are you breastfeeding your child? Are you giving him bottles? Milk in a cup? What kind of milk does he drink? How much?
- How much fruit juice or how many sweetened drinks (fruit drinks, soft drinks) does your child drink? Is the juice 100% fruit juice? When does he drink them?
- Which foods does your child like to eat? Are there any foods he doesn't like?
- Describe your child's mealtimes. Does he eat meals with the family?
- Does he ask for food between meals and snacks? If so, how do you handle this?
- Does your child throw tantrums over food? If so, how do you handle them?

Screening and Assessment

- Screen the child for lead exposure.
- Evaluate the child's progress in developing large motor skills. Children should be actively playing with a parent daily.

Anticipatory Guidance

Discuss With Parents

- Offering their child food every 2 to 3 hours. (Children's capacity to eat at any one time is limited.)
- Giving their child opportunities to develop eating skills (chewing, swallowing) by offering a variety of foods and eating at a family table.
- Providing forks and spoons designed for children (smaller and easier to use than utensils designed for adults).
- Turning off the television during mealtimes.
- Discouraging television viewing for children younger than age 2, and encouraging interactive activities (talking, playing, singing, and reading together).

2 YEARS

Interview Questions

- Has your child been weaned from the bottle?
- What kind of milk does she drink? How much?
- How much fruit juice or how many sweetened drinks (fruit drinks, soft drinks) does your child drink? Is the juice 100% fruit juice? When does she drink them?
- Which foods does your child like to eat? Are there any foods she doesn't like?

- Describe your child's mealtimes. How often does she eat with the family?
- Can your child shovel sand into a pail or pour water from a bucket? If she can, let her try to serve foods from a bowl or platter onto her plate.
- Does she eat the same foods as the rest of the family?

Screening and Assessment

- Screen the child for lead exposure.
- Assess the child's risk for familial hyperlipidemia.
- Evaluate the child's progress in developing large motor skills.

Anticipatory Guidance

Discuss With Parents

- Giving their child opportunities to develop eating skills (chewing, swallowing) by offering a variety of foods and eating at a family table.
- Allowing their child to self-regulate food intake by serving himself from bowls and plates. (This is messy at first, but with practice this self-help skill can be mastered.)
- Handling their child's food jags (wanting to eat only a particular food) by serving the favorite food along with other healthy foods.
- Turning off the television during mealtimes.

- Limiting total entertainment media time (watching television, playing computer or video games) to no more than 1 to 2 hours of quality programming a day.
- Encouraging interactive activities (talking, playing, singing, and reading together).

3 TO 4 YEARS

Interview Questions

- What kind of milk does your child drink? How much?
- How much fruit juice or how many sweetened drinks (fruit drinks, soft drinks) does your child drink? Is the juice 100% fruit juice? When does he drink them?
- Which foods does your child like to eat? Are there any foods he doesn't like?
- What concerns do you have about your child's weight?
- Describe what your child does during mealtimes. Does he serve himself foods? Does he eat meals with the family?
- How often do you serve snacks? What types of foods do you serve?

Screening and Assessment

- Screen the child for lead exposure.
- Obtain the child's blood pressure.
- Assess the child's risk for familial hyperlipidemia.

- Evaluate the child's progress in developing large motor skills. Children should be actively playing with a parent daily. By this age, many children can master running, marching, and galloping. Adults can direct children in ways to move their bodies around and through objects and in how to improve large and small muscle movements.

Anticipatory Guidance

Discuss With Parents

- Increasing their child's awareness of new foods by making sure the child sees family members and friends trying and enjoying them.
- Teaching their child about new foods by growing, preparing, and talking about them.
- Sharing stories, drawing pictures, and singing songs about food to help their child become familiar with them.
- Helping their child become more fit (stability, agility, endurance, and coordination).
- Turning off the television during mealtimes.
- Limiting total entertainment media time (watching television, playing computer or video games) to no more than 1 to 2 hours of quality programming a day.
- Encouraging interactive activities (talking, playing, singing, and reading together).

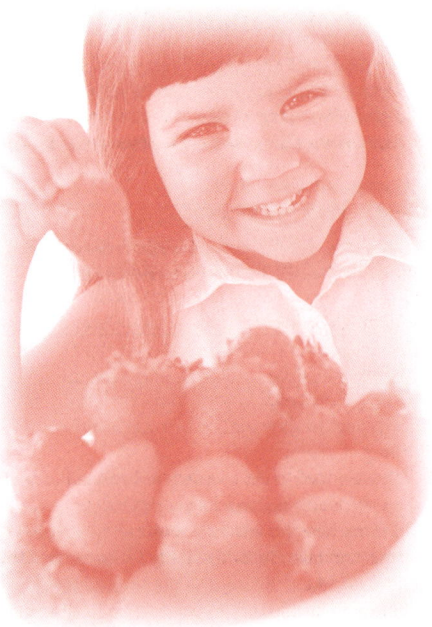

MIDDLE CHILDHOOD

OVERVIEW

Middle childhood, ages 5 to 10, is a period characterized by slow, steady physical growth. However, cognitive, emotional, and social development occur at a rapid pace.

Growth and Development

- Children in middle childhood gain an average of 7 lbs in weight and 2½ inches in height per year.
- Growth spurts, accompanied by increased appetite and food intake, are common. Conversely, appetite and food intake decrease during periods of slower growth.
- Body composition and body shape remain relatively constant.

Eating

- Children need to eat a variety of healthy foods. They need 3 meals plus 1 or 2 snacks per day.
- Children begin to describe foods according to color, shape, and quantity and classify foods as ones they like and don't like.
- Children may identify foods that are healthy but may not know why they are healthy.
- Children begin to realize that eating healthy food has a positive effect on growth and health.
- Children's ability to feed themselves improves, and they can help with simple food preparation and tasks related to mealtime.
- Mealtimes take on more social significance, and outside sources (peers, the media) begin to exert more influence over children's attitudes toward eating behaviors and food.
- Children's food intake is strongly associated with what their parents eat.

Body Image

- Children may become overly concerned about their physical appearance.
- Girls may be especially worried about being overweight and may begin to eat less or diet.
- Girls need to be reassured that increased body fat is part of normal growth and development and probably is not permanent.
- Boys may be concerned about their stature and muscle size and strength.
- During middle childhood, muscle-building activities (weight lifting) do not build muscle mass and can be harmful; muscle strength can be improved with appropriate physical activities.

Oral Health

- Children begin to lose primary teeth, and permanent teeth begin to erupt.
- Children may have difficulty chewing certain foods, such as raw vegetables or meat, if they are missing teeth or undergoing orthodontic treatment, and they may require foods that are easier to eat.

Physical Activity

- Children's muscle strength, motor skills, and stamina increase.
- Children acquire the motor skills required for complex movements, allowing them to engage in a variety of physical activities.
- Children are motivated to be physically active by having fun, feeling competent, and engaging in a variety of activities.
- Parents influence a child's level of physical activity when they participate with their child and show that physical activity is fun.
- Parents' encouragement to be physically active significantly increases their child's activity level.
- Teachers and children's friends influence a child's physical activity level.
- Participating in physical activity programs helps children learn to cooperate with others.

COMMON NUTRITION CONCERNS

- Decrease in consumption of milk and other milk products.
- Increase in consumption of sweetened beverages, especially soft drinks.
- Limited intake of fruits and vegetables.
- Higher consumption than recommended of foods high in fat, especially saturated and trans fats.
- Rise in overweight and obesity.
- Increase in body image concerns.

(See Key Indicators of Nutrition Risk for Children and Adolescents.)

NUTRITION SUPERVISION

A child's nutrition status should be evaluated during nutrition supervision visits or as part of health supervision visits. Health professionals can do the following:

- Begin nutrition supervision by selectively asking interview questions or by reviewing a questionnaire filled out by parents before the visit. Continue by conducting screening and assessment and providing anticipatory guidance.

- Recognize that interview questions, screening and assessment, and anticipatory guidance will vary from visit to visit and from child to child.
- See Strategies for Health Professionals to Promote Healthy Eating Behaviors.

Interview Questions

Eating Behaviors and Food Choices

For the Child

- Which meals do you usually eat each day? How many snacks?
- How often does your family eat meals together?
- Where did you eat yesterday? At school? At home? At a friend's house?
- What do you usually eat and drink in the morning? Around noon? In the afternoon? In the evening? Between meals?
- What snacks do you usually eat?
- What is your favorite food?
- Are there any foods you won't eat? If so, which ones?
- What do you usually drink with your meals? With snacks?
- What fruits and vegetables, including juices, did you eat or drink yesterday?

For the Parent

- How often does your family eat meals together?
- Do you have any concerns about your child's eating habits or behaviors (getting him to drink enough milk)?
- Do you think your child eats healthy foods? Why or why not?
- How often does your child eat breakfast?
- What does he usually eat for snacks?
- Where does your child eat snacks? At home? At school? At after-school care? At a friend's house?
- What does he usually drink (milk, water, fruit juice, fruit drinks, soft drinks)?

Food Resources

For the Child or Parent

- Who usually buys the food for your family? Who prepares it?
- Are there times when there is not enough food to eat or not enough money to buy food?

Weight and Body Image

For the Younger Child

- How do you feel about your weight?

For the Older Child

- How do you feel about your weight?
- How much would you like to weigh?
- Are you trying to change your weight? If so, how?

For the Parent

- How do you feel about your child's weight?

Physical Activity

For the Child

- What do you do to be physically active? How often?
- How much time do you spend being active in a week?
- How much time do you spend each day watching television and playing computer or video games?
- What do you think you can do to be more active?

For the Parent

- What types of physical activity does your child engage in? How often?
- How much time does your child spend each day watching television or playing computer or video games?
- Does your child have a television in his bedroom?

Screening and Assessment

Growth and Physical Development

- Measure the child's height and weight, and plot them on a standard growth chart. Deviation from expected growth patterns should be evaluated. This may be normal or may indicate a nutrition problem.
- Determine the child's nutrition status and overall health using body mass index (BMI). Calculate the child's BMI by dividing weight by square of height (kg/m^2), or use a BMI wheel or calculator. Plot the child's BMI and age on a BMI-for-age growth chart to determine BMI percentile.
- Evaluate the appearance of the child's skin, hair, teeth, gums, tongue, and eyes.
- Obtain the child's blood pressure.
- Assess the child's risk for familial hyperlipidemia.

Stunting

- If height-for-age is below the third percentile, evaluate to determine whether growth is stunted and whether the child may benefit from improved nutrition or treatment of other underlying problems.
- Low height-for-age is usually the result of genetics, not the result of stunted growth.

Underweight

- If BMI is below the fifth percentile, assess for organic disease and eating disorders.
- Children with a low BMI may be thin naturally or may be thin as a result of inadequate energy intake, inadequate food resources, restrictive dieting, a nutritional deficit, or a chronic disease.

Overweight and Obesity

- If BMI is between the 85th and 94th percentiles, the child is considered overweight and needs further screening.
- If BMI is at or above the 95th percentile, the child is considered obese and needs in-depth medical assessment.

Iron-Deficiency Anemia

Guidelines from the American Academy of Pediatrics (AAP) and the Centers for Disease Control and Prevention (CDC):

- Screen children consuming a strict vegetarian diet without iron supplementation. (AAP)
- Screen children with known risk factors for iron-deficiency anemia (low iron intake, special health care needs, previous diagnosis of iron-deficiency anemia). (CDC)

Oral Health

- Determine whether the child has regular dental visits.
- Assess eating behaviors (frequency of consuming foods and beverages high in sugar) to determine the child's risk for dental caries (tooth decay).

Physical Activity

- Determine how much physical activity the child engages in weekly. Compare the child's physical fitness level with national standards (school's standardized physical fitness assessment).
- Determine how much time the child spends watching television and on other media activities (computer, video games). Determine whether the child watches television during mealtimes.

Anticipatory Guidance

Discuss With Parents, the Child, or Both

Growth and Physical Development

- Expected accelerated growth (for girls at ages 9–11, for boys at about age 12).
- Variation in onset of puberty among children.
- Upcoming physical changes and specific concerns.

- How the child compares to others on a standard growth chart.
- Healthy body weight based on genetically determined size and shape rather than on socially defined ideal weight.
- Positive body image. (People come in unique sizes and shapes, within a range of healthy body weights.) (See Tips for Fostering a Positive Body Image Among Children and Adolescents.)
- Assuring children that they are loved and accepted as they are, regardless of their size and shape.
- Eating healthy foods and being physically active to achieve or maintain a healthy weight.
- Weight loss should not occur in children with BMI below the 95th percentile; gradual weight loss of no more than 1 lb per month may be appropriate for children with BMI between the 95th and 99th percentiles. A weight loss of no more than 2 lbs per week may be appropriate for children with BMI above the 99th percentile. (But, even if they are losing weight, children need to consume sufficient calories and nutrients for growth and development.)

Eating Behaviors and Food Choices

- Increasing the variety of foods the child eats and finding ways to incorporate new foods into the child's diet.
- Making healthy foods choices based on *Dietary Guidelines for Americans* (fruits, vegetables, grain products [especially whole grain]; low-fat [1%] and fat-free [skim] milk products [milk, cheese, yogurt]; and lean meats, poultry, fish, beans, eggs, and nuts).
- Energy requirements are influenced by growth, physical activity level, and body composition.
- Children ages 2 to 8 need to drink 2 cups of low-fat (1%) or fat-free (skim) milk per day or consume the equivalent from other milk products (cheese, yogurt).
- Children ages 9 and older need to drink 3 cups of low-fat (1%) or fat-free (skim) milk per day or consume the equivalent from other milk products.
- Providing a vitamin D supplement of 400 IU per day for children who do not obtain 400 IU per day of vitamin D through vitamin D–fortified milk (100 IU per 8-oz serving) and vitamin D–fortified foods (fortified cereals, eggs [yolks]).
- Eating 3 meals and 1 to 2 snacks per day.

- Choosing healthy foods for meals and snacks rich in complex carbohydrates (whole-grain products, fresh fruits and vegetables).
- Making family mealtimes a priority.
- Providing a relaxed atmosphere for mealtimes and getting rid of distractions (television).
- Limiting foods high in calories and low in nutrients.
- Limiting foods high in fat, especially high in saturated and trans fats (chips, french fries), and foods (candy, cookies) and beverages (fruit drinks, soft drinks) high in sugar.
- Enrolling child in school breakfast and lunch programs, if needed. (See Federal Nutrition Assistance Programs.)

Oral Health

- Toothbrushing requires good fine motor control, and young children cannot clean their teeth without help. (After children acquire fine motor skills [ability to tie their shoelaces], typically by age 7 or 8, they can brush their teeth effectively.)
- Brushing teeth with fluoridated toothpaste twice a day (after breakfast and before bed).
- Drinking water when thirsty.

- Using community fluoridated water as a safe, effective way to reduce dental caries. (If bottled water is preferred, recommend a brand with fluoride added at a concentration of approximately 0.8–1.0 mg/L [ppm].)
- Limiting foods (candy, cookies) and beverages (juice, juice drinks, soft drinks) high in sugar.

Physical Activity

- Engaging in 60 or more minutes of daily physical activity.
  - Aerobic: Either moderate-intensity (hiking, skateboarding) or vigorous-intensity (running, bicycling) aerobic physical activity daily, and include vigorous-intensity physical activity at least 3 days a week.
  - Muscle-strengthening: Include muscle-strengthening physical activity (climbing trees, sit-ups) at least 3 days a week.
  - Bone-strengthening: Include bone-strengthening (weight-bearing) physical activity (jumping rope, playing basketball) at least 3 days a week.
- For children with special health care needs, engaging in physical activity for cardiovascular fitness (within limits of medical or physical conditions).
- Wearing appropriate safety equipment (helmets, pads, mouth guards, goggles) when physically active.

- Drinking water when physically active. (Children are at increased risk for heat-related illness because their sweat glands are not fully developed.)
- Not having a television in the child's bedroom.
- Limiting total entertainment media time (watching television, playing computer or video games) to no more than 1 to 2 hours of quality programming a day.
- Reducing sedentary behaviors (watching television, playing computer or video games), especially if the child is overweight.

Substance Use

- Dangers of using alcohol, tobacco, and other drugs.
- Dangers of using performance-enhancing products (protein supplements, anabolic steroids).

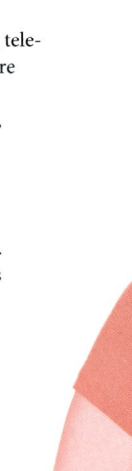

ADOLESCENCE

OVERVIEW

Adolescence is a period of dramatic physical, cognitive, social, and emotional changes. This developmental period is divided into 3 stages.

Early adolescence (ages 11–14). Adolescents are characterized by pubertal changes and a growing capacity for abstract thought, although concrete and oriented toward the present.

Middle adolescence (ages 15–17). Adolescents are characterized by independence, experimentation, future-oriented thinking, and problem-solving abilities.

Late adolescence (ages 18–21). This stage is a time of important personal and vocational decisions and refined abilities to reason logically and solve problems.

Growth and Development

- Adolescents achieve the final 15% to 20% of their adult height and gain 50% of their adult weight.
- Adolescents accumulate up to 40% of their skeletal mass.
- Nutrient needs are greatest during peak periods of growth (sexual maturity rating [SMR] 2–3 in females, 3–4 in males).
- Females complete most physical growth about 2 years after menarche. Mean age of menarche is 12.5 years.
- Males begin puberty about 2 years later than females.
- Males experience major growth spurts and increases in muscle mass during middle adolescence.
- Cognitive capacities increase dramatically during adolescence.
- Developing an identity and becoming an independent young adult are central to adolescence.

Eating

- Foods can have symbolic meanings. Adolescents may use them to establish individuality and express their identity.
- Adolescents may adopt certain eating behaviors (such as vegetarianism) to explore various lifestyles or to show concern for the environment.
- Interest in new foods, including those from different cultures and ethnic groups, is common during adolescence.
- Adolescents spend more time away from home and eat more meals and snacks away from home than when they were younger. Many adolescents go to stores and fast-food restaurants and purchase food with their own money.

Body Image

- Changes associated with puberty can affect adolescents' satisfaction with their appearance.
- For males, increased size and muscle development that come with physical maturation usually improve their body image.
- For females, physical maturation may lead to dissatisfaction with their bodies, which may result in weight concerns and dieting.
- Social pressure to be thin and the stigma of obesity can lead to unhealthy eating behaviors and a poor body image during adolescence.
- Adolescents may try fad diets and underestimate the associated health risks.

Physical Activity

- As adolescents grow and develop, their motor skills increase, providing more opportunities for engaging in physical activity.
- Physical activity usually occurs in group settings, and adolescents' engagement in physical activity may be influenced by peers.
- Parents influence an adolescent's physical activity level when they participate with the adolescent and show that physical activity is fun.
- Parents' encouragement to be physically active significantly increases adolescents' activity levels.

COMMON NUTRITION CONCERNS

- Decrease in consumption of milk and other milk products.
- Increase in consumption of beverages high in sugar, especially soft drinks and sports drinks.
- Insufficient intake of fruits and vegetables.
- Higher consumption than recommended of foods high in fat, especially saturated and trans fats, cholesterol, and sodium.
- Rise in overweight and obesity.
- Low levels of physical activity.
- Increase in eating disorders, body image concerns, dieting, and unsafe weight-loss methods.
- Prevalence of iron-deficiency anemia (in females).
- Prevalence of hyperlipidemia.
- Food insecurity among adolescents from families with low incomes.

(See Key Indicators of Nutrition Risk for Children and Adolescents.)

NUTRITION SUPERVISION

An adolescent's nutrition status should be evaluated during nutrition supervision visits or as part of health supervision visits. Health professionals can do the following:

- Begin nutrition supervision by selectively asking interview questions or by reviewing a questionnaire filled out by parents and/or the adolescent before the visit. Continue by conducting screening and assessment and providing anticipatory guidance.
- Recognize that interview questions, screening and assessment, and anticipatory guidance will vary from visit to visit and from adolescent to adolescent.

(See Strategies for Health Professionals to Promote Healthy Eating Behaviors.)

Interview Questions

Eating Behaviors and Food Choices

For the Adolescent

- Which meals do you usually eat each day? How many snacks? How many times a week do you eat breakfast? Lunch? Dinner?
- How often does your family eat meals together?
- What do you usually eat and drink in the morning? Around noon? In the afternoon? In the evening? Between meals?
- What snacks do you usually eat?
- Are there any foods you won't eat? If there are, which ones?
- How often do you drink milk? What kind of milk do you drink (whole milk, reduced-fat [2%], low-fat [1%], fat-free [skim] milk)? What other milk products do you like to eat?
- What fruits and vegetables, including juices, did you eat or drink yesterday?
- How often do you drink soft drinks, energy drinks, or sports drinks?
- What changes would you like to make in the way you eat?

For the Parent

- How often does your family eat meals together?
- Do you have any concerns about your teenager's eating behaviors?
- Do you think your teenager eats healthy foods? Why or why not?

Food Resources

For the Adolescent or Parent

- Who usually buys the food for your family? Who prepares it?
- Are there times when there is not enough food to eat or not enough money to buy food?

Weight and Body Image

For the Adolescent

- How do you feel about the way you look?
- Do you think that you weigh too little? Weigh too much? Are just the right weight? Why?
- How do you feel about your weight and height?
- Are you trying to change your weight? If so, how?
- How much would you like to weigh?
- Are you teased about your weight?

For the Parent

- How do you feel about your teenager's weight and height?

Physical Activity

For the Adolescent

- What do you do for physical activity? How often?
- How much time do you spend being active in a week?
- What physical activity would you like to do that you are not doing now? How can you make time for it?
- How much time do you spend each day watching television and playing computer or video games?
- What do you think you can do to be more active?

For the Parent

- What type of physical activity does your teenager engage in? How often?
- How much time does your teenager spend each day watching television or playing computer or video games?
- Does your teenager have a television in his bedroom?

Growth and Physical Development

- Measure the adolescent's height and weight, and plot them on a standard growth chart. Deviation from expected growth patterns should be evaluated. This may be normal or may indicate a nutrition problem.
- Determine the adolescent's nutrition status and overall health using body mass index (BMI). Calculate the adolescent's BMI by dividing weight by square of height (kg/m^2), or use a BMI wheel or calculator. Plot the adolescent's BMI and age on a BMI-for-age growth chart to determine BMI percentile.
- Evaluate appearance of the adolescent's skin, hair, teeth, gums, tongue, and eyes.
- Obtain the adolescent's blood pressure.
- Assess the adolescent's risk for familial hyperlipidemia.

Stunting

- If height-for-age is below the third percentile, evaluate to determine whether growth is stunted and whether the adolescent may benefit from improved nutrition or treatment of other underlying problems.
- Low height-for-age is usually the result of genetics, not the result of stunted growth.

Underweight

- If BMI is below the 5th percentile, assess for organic diseases and eating disorders.
- Adolescents with a low BMI may be thin naturally or may be thin as a result of inadequate energy intake, inadequate food resources, restrictive dieting, a nutritional deficit, or a chronic disease.

Overweight and Obesity

- If BMI is between the 85th and 94th percentiles, the adolescent is considered overweight and needs further screening.
- If BMI is at or above the 95th percentile, the adolescent is considered obese and needs in-depth medical assessment.

Iron-Deficiency Anemia

Guidelines from the American Academy of Pediatrics (AAP) and the Centers for Disease Control and Prevention (CDC):

- Screen females ages 12 to 21 during routine physical exams. (AAP)

- Screen females ages 12 to 21 with known risk factors for iron-deficiency anemia (extensive menstrual or other blood loss, low iron intake, previous diagnosis of iron-deficiency anemia) annually. For those with no known risk factors, screen every 5 to 10 years during routine physical examinations. (CDC)
- Screen males ages 12 to 18 during their peak growth period during routine physical examinations. (AAP)
- Screen males ages 12 to 18 with known risk factors for iron-deficiency anemia (low iron intake, special health care needs, previous diagnosis of iron-deficiency anemia). (CDC)

Oral Health

- Determine whether the adolescent has regular dental visits.
- Assess eating behaviors (frequency of consuming foods and beverages high in sugar) to determine the adolescent's risk for dental caries (tooth decay).

Physical Activity

- Determine how much physical activity the adolescent engages in weekly. Compare the adolescent's physical fitness level with national standards (school's standardized physical fitness assessment).

- Determine how much time the adolescent spends watching television and on other media activities (computer, video games). Determine whether the adolescent watches television during mealtimes.

Anticipatory Guidance

Discuss With Adolescent, Parents, or Both

Growth and Physical Development

- How the adolescent compares with others on the standard growth chart.
- Upcoming physical changes and specific concerns.
- For females, normal accumulation of fat in hips, thighs, and buttocks. (Fat accumulation ranges from 15%–18% of body weight before puberty to 20%–25% at the end of puberty.)
- For males, a slight weight gain before a growth spurt (between ages 9 and 13), a decrease in body fat during the growth spurt, and an increase in body fat after puberty (by age 18, about 15%–18% of body weight).
- For late-maturing males, ages 15 to 17, reassurance that their growth is normal. (Use charts that plot height velocity by age and SMR to ease concerns.)

Eating Behaviors and Food Choices

- Making healthy foods choices based on *Dietary Guidelines for Americans* (fruits, vegetables, grain products [especially whole grain]; low-fat [1%] and fat-free [skim] milk products [milk, cheese, yogurt]; and lean meats, poultry, fish, beans, eggs, and nuts).
- Drinking 3 cups of low-fat (1%) or fat-free (skim) milk per day or consuming the equivalent from other milk products (cheese, yogurt).
- Taking a vitamin D supplement of 400 IU per day for adolescents who do not obtain 400 IU per day of vitamin D through vitamin D–fortified milk (100 IU per 8-oz serving) and vitamin D–fortified foods (fortified cereals, eggs [yolk]).
- Eating 3 meals and snacks, as needed, per day.
- Limiting foods high in fat, especially high in saturated and trans fats (chips, french fries), and foods (candy, cookies) and beverages (fruit drinks, soft drinks) high in sugar.
- Enrolling adolescent in school breakfast and lunch programs, if needed. (See Federal Nutrition Assistance Programs.)

Oral Health

- Brushing teeth with fluoridated toothpaste twice a day (after breakfast and before bed).
- Drinking water when thirsty.
- Using community fluoridated water as a safe, effective way to reduce dental caries. (If bottled water is preferred, recommend a brand with fluoride added at a concentration of approximately 0.8–1.0 mg/L [ppm].)
- Limiting foods (candy, cookies) and beverages (juice, juice drinks, soft drinks) high in sugar.

Weight and Body Image

- Healthy body weight based on genetically determined size and shape rather than on socially defined ideal weight.
- Safe and healthy ways for achieving and maintaining healthy weight (practicing healthy eating behaviors; limiting high-calorie, low-nutrient foods and beverages; engaging in regular physical activity; reducing sedentary behaviors).
- Discouraging dieting; instead, emphasizing healthy lifestyle.

- Positive body image. (People come in unique sizes and shapes, within a range of healthy body weights.) (See Tips for Fostering a Positive Body Image Among Children and Adolescents.)
- Assuring adolescents that they are loved and accepted as they are, regardless of their size and shape.

Physical Activity

- Engaging in 60 or more minutes of daily physical activity.
  - Aerobic: Either moderate-intensity (hiking, skateboarding) or vigorous-intensity (running, bicycling) aerobic physical activity daily, and include vigorous-intensity physical activity at least 3 days a week.
  - Muscle-strengthening: Include muscle-strengthening physical activity (climbing trees, sit-ups) at least 3 days a week.
  - Bone-strengthening: Include bone-strengthening (weight-bearing) physical activity (jumping rope, playing basketball) at least 3 days a week.
- Incorporating physical activity into daily life (through physical education at school and activities with family and friends).
- For adolescents with special health care needs, engaging in physical activity for cardiovascular fitness (within limits of medical or physical conditions).

- Wearing appropriate safety equipment (helmets, pads, mouth guards, goggles) when physically active.
- Finding safe settings for physical activity.
- Drinking water when physically active.
- Not having a television in the adolescent's bedroom.
- Limiting total entertainment media time (watching television, playing computer or video games) to no more than 1 to 2 hours of quality programming a day.
- Reducing sedentary behaviors (watching television, playing computer or video games, especially if the adolescent is overweight.

Substance Use

- Consuming excessive quantities of caffeinated beverages (soft drinks, coffee, energy drinks).
- Dangers of using alcohol, tobacco, and other drugs.
- Dangers of using performance-enhancing products (protein supplements, anabolic steroids).

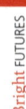

Nutrition Tools

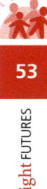

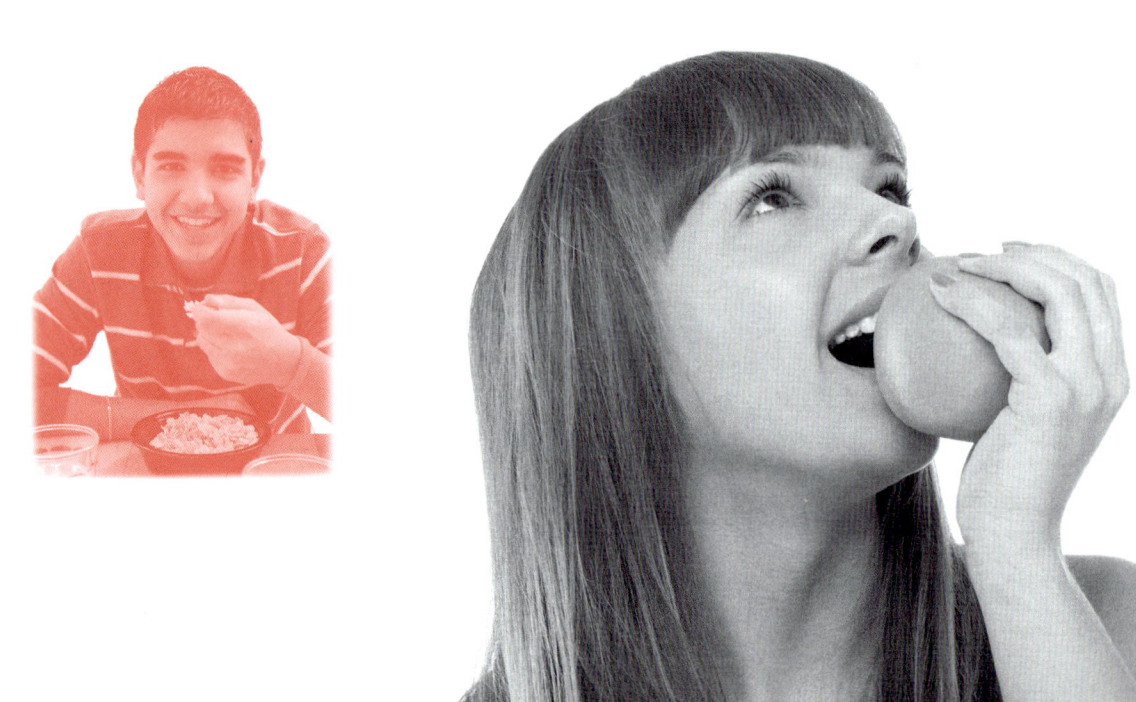

KEY INDICATORS OF NUTRITION RISK FOR CHILDREN AND ADOLESCENTS

INDICATORS OF NUTRITION RISK	RELEVANCE	CRITERIA FOR FURTHER SCREENING AND ASSESSMENT
Food Choices		
Consumes <2 servings of fruits per day. Consumes <3 servings of vegetables per day.	Fruits and vegetables provide vitamins (such as A and C), minerals, and fiber. Low intake of fruits and vegetables is associated with an increased risk of many types of cancer.	Assess the child or adolescent who is consuming <1 serving of fruit per day. Assess the child or adolescent who is consuming <2 servings of vegetables per day.
Consumes <6 servings of cereal, bread, crackers, pasta, rice, or other pasta per day. Consumes <3 servings of whole grains per day.	Grain products provide complex carbohydrates, vitamins, minerals, and fiber. Low intake of fiber is associated with constipation and increased risk of colon cancer.	Assess the child or adolescent who is consuming <6 servings of cereal, bread, crackers, rice, pasta, or other grains per day. Assess the child or adolescent who is consuming <3 servings of whole-grain cereal, bread, crackers, rice, pasta, or other grains per day. Assess the child or adolescent who has recent history of constipation.

KEY INDICATORS OF NUTRITION RISK FOR CHILDREN AND ADOLESCENTS, CONTINUED

INDICATORS OF NUTRITION RISK	RELEVANCE	CRITERIA FOR FURTHER SCREENING AND ASSESSMENT
Food Choices, continued		
For children <9: Consumes <2 servings of milk and milk products per day. For children ≥9 and adolescents: Consumes <3 servings of milk and milk products per day.	Milk and milk products are a good source of protein, vitamins, and calcium and other minerals. Low intake of milk and milk products may reduce peak bone mass and increase the risk of osteoporosis.	Assess the child (<9) who is consuming <1 serving of milk and milk products per day. Assess the child (≥9) or adolescent who is consuming <2 servings of milk and milk products per day. Assess the child or adolescent who has a milk allergy or is lactose intolerant. Assess the child or adolescent who is consuming >2 soft drinks per day.

KEY INDICATORS OF NUTRITION RISK FOR CHILDREN AND ADOLESCENTS, CONTINUED

INDICATORS OF NUTRITION RISK	RELEVANCE	CRITERIA FOR FURTHER SCREENING AND ASSESSMENT
Consumes <2 servings of meat or meat alternatives (eg, beans, eggs, nuts, seeds) per day.	Protein-rich foods (eg, meats, meat alternatives) are good sources of B vitamins, iron, and zinc. Low intake of protein-rich foods may impair growth and increase the risk of iron-deficiency anemia and of delayed growth and sexual maturation. Low intake of meat or meat alternatives may indicate inadequate availability of these foods at home. Special attention should be paid to children and adolescents who follow a vegetarian diet.	Assess the child or adolescent who is consuming <1 serving of meat or meat alternatives per day.
For children ≥5: Consumes excessive amount of fat.	Excessive intake of dietary fat contributes to the risk of cardiovascular disease and obesity and is associated with some cancers.	Assess the child or adolescent who has a family history of premature cardiovascular disease. Assess the child or adolescent if body mass index (BMI) is ≥85th percentile.

KEY INDICATORS OF NUTRITION RISK FOR CHILDREN AND ADOLESCENTS, CONTINUED

INDICATORS OF NUTRITION RISK	RELEVANCE	CRITERIA FOR FURTHER SCREENING AND ASSESSMENT
Eating Behaviors		
Exhibits poor appetite.	A poor appetite may be developmentally appropriate for young children, but in older children and adolescents it may indicate depression or other emotional stress, or a chronic disease.	Assess the child or adolescent if BMI is <15th percentile or if weight loss has occurred. Assess the child or adolescent if irregular menses or amenorrhea has occurred for ≥3 months. Assess the child or adolescent for organic and psychiatric disease.
Consumes food from fast-food restaurants ≥3 times per week.	Excessive consumption of convenience foods and foods from fast-food restaurants is associated with high fat, calorie, and sodium intake, as well as low intake of certain vitamins and minerals.	Assess the child or adolescent who is overweight or obese or who has diabetes mellitus, hyperlipidemia, or other conditions requiring reduction in dietary fat.

KEY INDICATORS OF NUTRITION RISK FOR CHILDREN AND ADOLESCENTS, CONTINUED

INDICATORS OF NUTRITION RISK	RELEVANCE	CRITERIA FOR FURTHER SCREENING AND ASSESSMENT
Skips breakfast, lunch, or dinner or supper ≥3 times per week.	Meal-skipping is associated with a low intake of energy and essential nutrients and, if it is a regular practice, could compromise growth and development. Repeatedly skipping meals decreases the nutritional adequacy of the diet.	Assess the child or adolescent to ensure that meal-skipping is not due to inadequate food resources or unhealthy weight-loss practices.
Has food jags—eats one particular food only.	Food jags, which limit the variety of food consumed, decrease the nutritional adequacy of the diet.	Assess the child's or adolescent's dietary intake over several days.
Food Resources		
Has inadequate financial resources to buy food, insufficient access to food, or lack of access to cooking facilities.	Poverty can result in hunger and compromised food quality and nutrition status. Inadequate dietary intake interferes with learning.	Assess the child or adolescent who is from a family with low income, is homeless, or is a runaway.

KEY INDICATORS OF NUTRITION RISK FOR CHILDREN AND ADOLESCENTS, CONTINUED

INDICATORS OF NUTRITION RISK	RELEVANCE	CRITERIA FOR FURTHER SCREENING AND ASSESSMENT
Weight and Body Image		
Practices unhealthy behaviors (eg, chronic dieting, vomiting; and using laxatives, diuretics, or diet pills to lose weight).	Chronic dieting is associated with many health concerns (eg, fatigue, impaired growth and sexual maturation, irritability, poor concentration, impulse to binge) and can lead to eating disorders. Frequent dieting in combination with purging is associated with health-compromising behaviors (eg, substance use, suicidal behaviors). Purging is associated with serious medical complications.	Assess the child or adolescent for eating disorders. Assess the child or adolescent for organic and psychiatric disease.
Is excessively concerned about body size or shape.	Eating disorders are associated with significant health and psychosocial morbidity. Eighty-five percent of all cases of eating disorders begin during adolescence. The earlier adolescents are treated, the better their long-term prognosis.	Assess the child or adolescent for distorted body image and dysfunctional eating behaviors, especially if the child or adolescent wants to lose weight but BMI is <85th percentile.

INDICATORS OF NUTRITION RISK	RELEVANCE	CRITERIA FOR FURTHER SCREENING AND ASSESSMENT
Exhibits significant weight change in past 6 months.	Significant weight change during the past 6 months may indicate stress, depression, organic disease, or an eating disorder.	Assess the child or adolescent to determine the cause of weight loss or weight gain (eg, limited or too much access to food, poor appetite, meal-skipping, eating disorder).
Growth		
Has BMI <5th percentile.	Thinness may indicate an eating disorder or poor nutrition.	Assess the child or adolescent for eating disorders. Assess the child or adolescent for organic or psychiatric disease. Assess the child or adolescent for inadequate food resources.
Has BMI >85th percentile.	Overweight children and adolescents are more likely to be overweight adults and are at increased risk for health problems as adults. Obesity is associated with elevated cholesterol levels and elevated blood pressure. Obesity is an independent risk factor for cardiovascular disease and type 2 diabetes mellitus.	Assess the child or adolescent who is at risk for overweight.

KEY INDICATORS OF NUTRITION RISK FOR CHILDREN AND ADOLESCENTS, CONTINUED

INDICATORS OF NUTRITION RISK	RELEVANCE	CRITERIA FOR FURTHER SCREENING AND ASSESSMENT
Physical Activity		
Is physically inactive: participates in physical activity <5 days per week.	Lack of physical activity is associated with overweight and obesity, fatigue, and poor muscle tone in the short term and a greater risk of cardiovascular disease in the long term. Regular physical activity reduces the risk of cardiovascular disease, hypertension, colon cancer, and type 2 diabetes mellitus. Weight-bearing physical activity is essential for normal skeletal development during childhood. Regular physical activity is necessary for maintaining normal muscle strength, joint structure, and joint function; contributes to psychological health and well-being; and facilitates weight reduction and weight maintenance throughout life.	Assess how much time the child or adolescent spends watching television or DVDs and playing computer games. Assess the child's or adolescent's definition of physical activity.

KEY INDICATORS OF NUTRITION RISK FOR CHILDREN AND ADOLESCENTS, CONTINUED

INDICATORS OF NUTRITION RISK	RELEVANCE	CRITERIA FOR FURTHER SCREENING AND ASSESSMENT
Participates in excessive physical activity.	Intense physical activity nearly every day, sometimes more than once a day, can be unhealthy and may be associated with menstrual irregularity, excessive weight loss, and malnutrition.	Assess the child or adolescent for eating disorders.
Lifestyle		
Engages in heavy alcohol, tobacco, and other drug use.	Alcohol, tobacco, and other drug use can adversely affect nutrient intake and nutrition status.	Assess the child or adolescent further for alcohol, tobacco, and other drug use.
Uses dietary supplements.	Dietary supplements (eg, vitamin and mineral preparations) can be healthy additions to a diet for children or adolescents with a history of iron-deficiency anemia; however, high doses can have serious side effects. Adolescents who use supplements to "bulk up" may be tempted to experiment with anabolic steroids.	Assess the child or adolescent for the type of supplements used and dosage. Assess adolescent's use of anabolic steroids and mega doses of other supplements.

63

STRATEGIES FOR HEALTH PROFESSIONALS TO PROMOTE HEALTHY EATING BEHAVIORS

STRATEGIES	APPLICATIONS/QUESTIONS
Communication Factors	
Promote positive, nonjudgmental strategies to help the child or adolescent adopt healthy eating behaviors.	Reinforce positive aspects of the child's or adolescent's eating behaviors.
Encourage the child's or adolescent's active participation in changing eating behaviors.	Help the child or adolescent identify barriers that make it difficult to change eating behaviors, and develop a plan of action for adopting new behaviors.
Provide concrete learning situations.	Use charts, food models, and videotapes to reinforce verbal information and instructions.
Focus on the short-term benefits of healthy eating behaviors.	Emphasize that healthy eating behaviors will make the child or adolescent feel good and have more energy.
Understand and respect the child's or adolescent's cultural eating behaviors.	Help the child or adolescent integrate cultural eating behaviors with dietary recommendations.
Use simple terminology.	Avoid using the term "diet" with the child or adolescent because it tends to be associated with weight loss and may be confusing.

STRATEGIES FOR HEALTH PROFESSIONALS TO PROMOTE HEALTHY EATING BEHAVIORS, CONTINUED

STRATEGIES	APPLICATIONS/QUESTIONS
Environmental Factors	
Create an office or clinic environment oriented to children or adolescents.	Use posters and materials written for children or adolescents.
Communicate developmentally appropriate health messages.	Use posters and materials that highlight the importance of healthy eating behaviors.
Encourage health professionals and staff to become role models for healthy eating behaviors.	Have health professionals and staff model healthy eating behaviors.
Readiness to Change	
Identify the child's or adolescent's stage of behavior change and readiness to change based on the Stages of Change model (Tool F in *Bright Futures: Nutrition* manual).	"Do you want to change the way you eat?" "Are you thinking about changing the way you eat?" "Are you ready to change the way you eat?" "Are you changing the way you eat?" "Are you trying to keep eating the way you have been?"
Facilitate behavior change with counseling strategies tailored to the child or adolescent based on the Stages of Change model (Tool F in *Bright Futures: Nutrition* manual).	Provide a supportive environment, basic information, and assessment. Prioritize behaviors to be changed, set goals, and identify barriers to change. Develop a plan that incorporates incremental steps for making changes, support, and reinforcement.

STRATEGIES FOR HEALTH PROFESSIONALS TO PROMOTE HEALTHY EATING BEHAVIORS, CONTINUED

STRATEGIES	APPLICATIONS/QUESTIONS
Action Plans	
Provide counseling for the child or adolescent who is in the early stages of behavior change or who is unwilling to change.	Increase the child's or adolescent's awareness and knowledge of eating behaviors. Encourage the child or adolescent to make behavior changes.
Provide task-oriented counseling for the child or adolescent who is ready to change eating behaviors.	Encourage a few small, concrete changes first, and build on those. Support and follow up with the child or adolescent who has changed behavior.
Identify and prioritize behavior changes to be made.	Suggest changes that will have a measurable impact on the child's or adolescent's most serious nutrition issues.
Set realistic, achievable goals that are supported by the child's or adolescent's family.	"What will you change?" "What goal is realistic right now?" "How and when will you change, and who will help you?"
Identify and address barriers to behavior change; help reduce barriers when possible.	"What could make it hard for you to make this change—money, friends, or family?" "How can you get around this?"

STRATEGIES FOR HEALTH PROFESSIONALS TO PROMOTE HEALTHY EATING BEHAVIORS, CONTINUED

STRATEGIES	APPLICATIONS/QUESTIONS
Make sure that the behavior changes are compatible with the child's or adolescent's lifestyle.	Don't expect the child or adolescent to conform to rigid eating behaviors. Keep in mind current behaviors and realistic goals.
Establish incremental steps to help the child or adolescent change eating behaviors.	For example, have the child or adolescent reduce fat consumption by changing the type of milk consumed, from reduced-fat (2%), to low-fat (1%), to fat-free (skim) milk.
Encourage the child or adolescent to commit to behavior changes with contracts.	Discuss nonfood rewards (incentives) to help the child or adolescent focus on changing eating behaviors.
Give the child or adolescent responsibility for changing and monitoring eating behaviors.	Stress the importance of planning how the child or adolescent will make and track changes in eating behavior. Make record-keeping simple, and review the plan with the child or adolescent.
Help the child or adolescent obtain family and peer support.	Discuss how the child or adolescent can encourage parents and peers to help. Meet with parents to clarify goals and action plans; determine how they can help. Provide nutrition education or counseling to parents, as appropriate.

STRATEGIES FOR HEALTH PROFESSIONALS TO PROMOTE HEALTHY EATING BEHAVIORS, CONTINUED

STRATEGIES	APPLICATIONS/QUESTIONS
Offer feedback and reinforce successes.	Show interest to encourage continued behavior change.
General Strategies	
Ask the child or adolescent about changes in eating behaviors at every visit.	"How are you doing in changing the way you eat?"
Emphasize to the child or adolescent the consumption of foods rather than nutrients.	For example, say, "drink more milk, and eat more cheese, and yogurt" rather than "you need more calcium."
Build on positive aspects of the child's or adolescent's eating behaviors.	"It's great that you're eating breakfast. Would you be willing to try cereal, fruit, and toast instead of bacon and doughnuts 4 days a week?"
Focus on "how to" instead of "why" information.	Share behaviorally oriented information (eg, what, how much, and when to eat and how to prepare food) rather than focusing on why the information is important.
Provide counseling that integrates realistic behavior change into the child's or adolescent's lifestyle.	"I understand that your friends eat lunch at fast-food restaurants. Would it help you to learn how to make healthier food choices at these restaurants?"
Discuss how to make healthy food choices in a variety of settings.	Talk about how to choose foods in various settings such as fast-food and other restaurants, convenience stores, vending machines, and friends' homes.

STRATEGIES FOR HEALTH PROFESSIONALS TO PROMOTE HEALTHY EATING BEHAVIORS, CONTINUED

STRATEGIES	APPLICATIONS/QUESTIONS
Provide the child or adolescent with learning experiences and skills practice.	Practice problem-solving and role-playing (eg, having the child or adolescent ask the food server to hold the mayonnaise).
Introduce the concept of achieving balance and enjoying all foods in moderation.	"Your food record shows that after having pepperoni pizza for lunch yesterday, you ate a lighter dinner. That's a good way to balance your food intake throughout the day."
Make recordkeeping easy, and tell the child or adolescent that you do not expect spelling, handwriting, and eating behaviors to be perfect.	"Be as accurate and honest as you can as you record your food intake. This record is a tool to help you think about how you eat."
Make sure that the child or adolescent hears what you are saying.	"What are you planning to work on before your next appointment?"
Make sure that you and the child or adolescent define terms in the same way to avoid confusion.	Discuss the definition of words that may cause confusion, such as "fat," "calories," "meal," and "snack."
When assessing food intake, keep in mind that a child's or adolescent's portion size may not be the same as a standard serving size.	Use food models or household cups and bowls to clarify serving sizes.

Nutrition Tools

Bright FUTURES

TIPS FOR FOSTERING A POSITIVE BODY IMAGE AMONG CHILDREN AND ADOLESCENTS

CHILD OR ADOLESCENT	PARENTS	HEALTH PROFESSIONAL
Look in the mirror and focus on your positive features, not your negative ones. Say something nice to your friends about how they look. Think about your positive traits that are not related to appearance. Look at magazines with a critical eye, and find out what photographers and graphic designers do to make models look the way they do. If you are overweight and want to lose weight, be realistic in your expectations, and aim for gradual change. Realize that everyone has a unique size and shape. If you have questions about your size or weight, ask a health professional.	Model healthy eating and physical activity behaviors, and avoid extreme eating and physical activity behaviors. Focus on non–appearance-related traits when discussing yourself and others. Praise your child or adolescent for academic and other successes. Analyze media messages with your child or adolescent. Show that you love your child or adolescent regardless of what he weighs. If your child or adolescent is overweight, don't criticize her appearance—offer support instead. Share with a health professional any concerns you have about your child's or adolescent's eating behaviors or body image.	Discuss changes that occur during adolescence. Assess weight concerns and body image. If a child or adolescent has a distorted body image, explore causes and discuss potential consequences. Discuss how the media negatively affects body image. Discuss normal variation in body sizes and shapes among children and adolescents. Educate parents, physical education instructors, and coaches about realistic and healthy body weights. Emphasize the positive characteristics (related to appearance and not related to appearance) of children and adolescents you see. Take extra time with an overweight child or adolescent to discuss psychosocial concerns and weight control options. Refer children, adolescents, and parents with weight-control issues to a registered dietitian or other health professional.

BASICS FOR HANDLING FOOD SAFELY[a]

Safe food handling, cooking, and storage are essential to prevent foodborne illness. You can't see, smell, or taste harmful bacteria that may cause illness. In every step of food preparation, follow 4 guidelines to keep food safe:

- Clean—Wash hands and surfaces often.
- Separate—Don't cross-contaminate.
- Cook—Cook to proper temperatures.
- Chill—Refrigerate promptly.

Shopping

- Buy refrigerated or frozen items after selecting non-perishable food.
- Never buy meat or poultry in packaging that is torn or leaking.
- Never buy food after "sell-by," "use-by," or other expiration dates.

Storage

- Always refrigerate perishable food within 2 hours (1 hour when the temperature is above 90° F).
- Check the temperatures of your refrigerator and freezer with an appliance thermometer. The refrigerator should be at 40°F or below and the freezer at 0°F or below.
- Cook or freeze fresh poultry, fish, ground meat, and variety meat (eg, calf's tongue) within 2 days; cook or freeze other beef, veal, lamb, or pork within 3 to 5 days.
- Make sure perishable food such as meat and poultry is wrapped securely to maintain quality and to prevent meat juices from coming into contact with other food.
- To maintain quality when freezing meat and poultry in its original package, wrap the package again with foil or plastic wrap that is recommended for the freezer.
- In general, canned high-acid foods such as tomatoes, grapefruit, and pineapple can be stored for 12 to 18 months. Canned low-acid foods such as meat, poultry, fish, and most vegetables can be stored for 2 to 5 years if the can remains in good condition and has been kept in a cool, clean, and dry place. Discard cans that are dented, leaking, bulging, or rusted.

BASICS FOR HANDLING FOOD SAFELY, CONTINUED

Preparation

- Always wash your hands with warm water and soap for 20 seconds before and after handling food.
- Don't cross-contaminate. Keep raw meat, poultry, fish, and their juices away from other food. After cutting raw meat, wash the cutting board, utensils, and countertops with hot, soapy water.
- Sanitize cutting boards, utensils, and countertops with a solution of 1 tablespoon of unscented, liquid chlorine bleach in 1 gallon of water.
- Marinate meat and poultry in a covered dish in the refrigerator.

Thawing

- Refrigerator: The refrigerator allows slow, safe thawing. Make sure thawing meat and poultry juices do not drip onto other food.
- Cold water: For faster thawing, place food in a leak-proof plastic bag, and submerge the bag in cold tap water. Change the water every 30 minutes. Cook immediately after thawing.
- Microwave: For fastest thawing, use the microwave. Place food in cookware that is manufactured for use in the microwave and cover with a lid or microwave-safe plastic wrap to hold in moisture and provide safe, even heating. Cook meat, poultry, egg casseroles, and fish immediately after microwave thawing.

Cooking (Minimal Internal Temperature)

- Beef, veal, and lamb steaks; roasts; and chops cooked to 145°F.
- All cuts of pork cooked to 160°F.
- Ground beef, veal, and lamb cooked to 160°F.
- Poultry cooked to 165°F.

BASICS FOR HANDLING FOOD SAFELY, CONTINUED

Serving

- Hot food should be held at 140°F or warmer.
- Cold food should be held at 40°F or colder.
- At buffets, keep food hot with chafing dishes, slow cookers, and warming trays. Keep food cold by nesting dishes in bowls of ice.
- Perishable food should not be kept at room temperature for more than 2 hours (1 hour when the temperature is above 90°F).

Leftovers

- Discard any perishable food kept at room temperature for more than 2 hours (1 hour if the temperature was above 90°F).
- Place perishable food in shallow containers and immediately put it in the refrigerator or freezer for rapid cooling.
- Use cooked leftovers within 4 days.

Refreezing

- Meat and poultry defrosted in the refrigerator may be refrozen before or after cooking. For meat thawed by other methods, cook before refreezing.

*Adapted from US Department of Agriculture, Food Safety and Inspection Service. *Basics for Handling Food Safely.* Washington, DC. US Department of Agriculture, Food Safety and Inspection Service; 2006.

FEDERAL NUTRITION ASSISTANCE PROGRAMS

FOOD ASSISTANCE AND NUTRITION PROGRAMS	SERVICES AND BENEFITS	WHO QUALIFIES	FUNDING AND ADMINISTRATIVE AGENCIES	SERVICE PROVIDERS
Child and Adult Care Food Program (CACFP)	Reduced-price or free meals and snacks	Children and adolescents up to age 12; children and adolescents up to age 15 from families of migrant workers; children and adolescents up to age 18 who are residents of emergency shelters; and children and adolescents with a disability (as defined by the state) enrolled in an institution, child care facility, or emergency shelter	US Department of Agriculture (USDA) State education agencies	Child care centers, day care homes, "at-risk" after-school care programs, and emergency shelters
Commodity Supplemental Food Program (CSFP)	Food	Infants and children up to age 6 from families with incomes at or <185% of the federal poverty level	USDA State agency (eg, health)	Local public and nonprofit private agencies

FEDERAL NUTRITION ASSISTANCE PROGRAMS, CONTINUED

FOOD ASSISTANCE AND NUTRITION PROGRAMS	SERVICES AND BENEFITS	WHO QUALIFIES	FUNDING AND ADMINISTRATIVE AGENCIES	SERVICE PROVIDERS
Early Head Start and Head Start	Nutrition services and meals and snacks (through the National School Lunch Program and the School Breakfast Program)	Infants and children up to age 5 and their families receiving public assistance or with incomes <100% of the federal poverty level; at least 10% of total enrollment available for infants and children with disabilities	Department of Health and Human Services (DHHS) DHHS regional offices	Local public and private nonprofit and for-profit agencies
The Emergency Food Assistance Program (TEFAP)	Food	Varies by state	USDA State agency	Local public and nonprofit private agencies (eg, food banks, food pantries, soup kitchens)
Expanded Food and Nutrition Education Program (EFNEP)	Nutrition education	Children and adolescents from families with limited resources	USDA State land grant universities and Cooperative Extension Service offices	Local Cooperative Extension Service offices

Bright FUTURES

FEDERAL NUTRITION ASSISTANCE PROGRAMS, CONTINUED

FOOD ASSISTANCE AND NUTRITION PROGRAMS	SERVICES AND BENEFITS	WHO QUALIFIES	FUNDING AND ADMINISTRATIVE AGENCIES	SERVICE PROVIDERS
Food Distribution Programs on Indian Reservations (FDPIR)	Food	Children and adolescents from families living on Indian reservations and children and adolescents from Native American families residing in designated areas near reservations and in the state of Oklahoma with a family member who belongs to a federally recognized tribe; eligibility based on income and resource standards	USDA Indian tribal organizations and USDA, Food and Nutrition office	Indian tribes and tribal organizations
National School Lunch Program (NSLP)	Reduced-price or free lunches and afternoon snacks	Children and adolescents attending school: reduced-price lunches and snacks are available if family income is between 130% and 185% of federal poverty level; free lunches and snacks are available if income is at or <130% of federal poverty level	USDA State education agencies	Public and private nonprofit schools and residential child care institutions